D1554624

This Shouldn't Hurt a Bit

Finding the Right IV Therapy For You

Bob Wheeler, Jr.

Table of Contents

INTRODUCTION

IV therapy is becoming trendy. It's becoming popular. Celebrities swear by it, and athletes preach about its miraculous effects. You've read basic claims from "feeling better" to preposterous notions of curing everything from Diabetes to Fibromyalgia, and might have been told it's the fountain of youth for everyone. Cancer treatment, weight loss, energy boost, and hair regrowth are a few of the ads you've likely seen, and the list goes on and on.

Can IV treatments really do all of these things? Can they do ANY of them? That's what we're here to explore.

Moreover, it seems these days that you can get an IV on every corner. From your family physician to your chiropractor, every healthcare practitioner is adding IVs as a service. And, it's not just medical professionals offering them. Everyone, up to and including your hair dresser, is making a go at offering you IV therapy.

No advertisement, no matter how slick or convincing, means IV therapy is right for you, or that you're getting it at the right place if it is. Nearly anyone can buy the supplies to give you an IV and find a doctor to sign the prescription, but being able to buy the IV catheter and the fluids doesn't mean someone is qualified to administer an IV safely, or that they're giving you what you need.

In this book we're going to explore the exploding world of IV therapy, its benefits and risks, find out if it's right for you, discuss what it can and can't do for you, tell you what to seek and what to avoid, and give you some tips on discovering where you can safely receive IV therapy.

Remember as you read this book that IV therapy is a serious medical procedure. Sure, it's relatively painless. Yes, you can get some treatments without lab work or a long doctor's appointment. You can take a nap or watch TV in a lounge chair while you're getting it. None of that convenience or luxury changes the fact that you are allowing someone to insert a needle into your vein and infuse compounds directly into your bloodstream. If you don't know why you're getting an IV, what you're getting, what the potential risks are, or who you're getting it from and what their commitment is, you're putting yourself at risk.

If you take care to find the right facility, go for the right reasons, and take an active part in your IV experience, it shouldn't hurt a bit.

CHAPTER 1:

Do You *NEED* IV Therapy?

Let's start off with "probably not", and go from there.

It's a lot easier to discuss the folks who really do need IV therapy than it is to list everyone who doesn't.

You can probably safely assume that if you don't fall into one of these categories, you don't REALLY *need* IV therapy. If you get something innocuous from a reputable provider, it certainly can't hurt to get an IV, but it might not be necessary.

1. You're DEHYDRATED

Simple dehydration is the number one reason to receive IV therapy in a non-urgent care or non-hospital setting. There are many others, but the basic reason to receive hydration intravenously at an IV therapy center/bar/spa is that your body simply doesn't have the fluids it requires to operate effectively, and the quickest, most effective way to hydrate is with an IV. You need fluids, but you don't want to sit in an ER waiting room with screaming Jimmy who broke his arm riding a skateboard, or sit in the lobby while the entire team at Quick Care is worried about Mr. Jones' potential heart attack. You also don't want to pay those massive bills. Still, you need more than just a few lemon-lime flavored sports drinks to get you right.

Though estimates vary, most studies (including those by the National Institute of Health and the University of Florida) show that somewhere between sixty to seventy-five percent of all Americans are chronically dehydrated. Chronically basically means "all the time". So, there's about a three in four chance you're dehydrated right now. Maybe you aren't dangerously dehydrated, but you aren't at peak hydration by any stretch. A simple anecdotal test of this is to look at your urine stream. If it's anything other than clear, you aren't taking in enough fluids, specifically water.

You're probably saying "so what" right about now. You feel fine. You don't have kidney stones, you aren't in a fog, don't have a throbbing headache, and you don't have badly chapped lips. If you seem to be getting by, what's a little dehydration going to really mean?

Remember, about 75% of your body weight is water. It's not just "in" your system, like tap-water in your stomach or veins, it "IS" your system. Your cells are comprised mostly of good old H_2O. Think of a basketball or football, or even tire, that doesn't have enough air in it. Your car has a warning system that your tire is low on air pressure. Sadly, by the time your body warns you that your cells are low on water, you've got a problem.

Dehydration, even mild dehydration, can cause some nasty problems in the body. The first few are obvious, like dry mouth, chapped lips, and chafed skin. A little dry mouth never killed anyone though right? Charles P. Davis, MD, PhD notes in his 2019 WebMD article on dehydration that though these symptoms are relatively innocuous, and may appear only to indicate mild dehydration, they're also the first signs of potentially hazardous dehydration. By the time you've added headache (or migraine) to your list of "mild" symptoms, you may well be on your way to severe dehydration.

To say the least, severe dehydration is another matter all-together. At this point you're looking at potential muscle cramping, kidney stones, dizziness, confusion, rapid heart rate (tachycardia), blood pressure swings, and possibly shock. In dramatic cases comas can occur.

Now that you're good and scared about dehydration, here's the good news: it's very easily prevented and cured.

Dr. Jack Dybis of IVme in Chicago has a simple formula for staying hydrated, and preventing the symptoms of dehydration. He says that you should take your weight in pounds, divide it in half, and drink that number of ounces of water per day. So, let's say you weigh 150 pounds. 150/2 is 75, so you need roughly 75 ounces of water a day according to the hydration expert doctor, or about five of the 16 ounce bottles of water.

But wait, what if you're past that point? What if you're already experiencing dehydration? Mild dehydration is something on which you can "catch up". Remember, water in your body isn't like gas in your car, where you are fine until you're out and then it dies, it's more like oil in your car, where not having enough can lead to problems, but doesn't lead to instant conking out. Slowly but steadily drinking lukewarm water can help immediately. As you no doubt remember from junior high science class, warm things cause expansion, and cold things cause contraction. That being the case you'll want to stay away from cold water because it will cause vasoconstriction (contraction of the venous system) which can lead to worsening symptoms of headache or cramping. Plain lukewarm water can be a near instant help. Drink it slowly but consistently until the first bottle or glass is gone, and then move on to cooler water for comfort.

The problem with "make-up" hydration is that just like driving around with too little oil in your car, once you've caused problems, you've got problems. A cycle of dehydration and rehydration is hell on your organs, cells, and tissue. Better to keep that water meter in the green all the time.

Unfortunately, life sometimes gets in the way of your glorious health plans. You decided 3k into the 5k that you were going to do the whole 10k. You got out on the boat and fell asleep in the sun. Your dog knocked over your tumbler full of water but you stayed outside and finished the entire yard anyway. Your softball team ended up in a three way tie at the top of the bracket and you had to play two more games. Lots of simple issues lead to dehydration that sometimes can't be fixed with a 32 ounce cup of water.

Long-term, sustained water drinking will keep you hydrated, but it takes several hours for your body to process even a half a liter (500ml) of water. Much of the water you drink is absorbed by your lips, mouth and tongue, and the rest must travel through your stomach, intestines, etc., before it can be put to use in your body. If you're two to three liters low on water (pretty standard) you can still be dehydrated after six hours of consistent drinking.

Worse, when your body is dehydrated it's not just lacking water, it's lacking the electrolytic components (electrolytes) that perform functions like allowing information to pass across neural pathways and creating the fuel for cellular function.

That's where the IV comes into play.

It generally takes between 35 minutes and one hour for the average person to absorb one full liter of fluids intravenously. The actual time of course depends on your level of dehydration, your overall fitness level, the size and health of your veins, and other factors. A young football player with great veins and a stellar physique may absorb an entire liter in 35 to 40 minutes, whereas the rest of us may take a little longer.

The important thing to note here isn't just that you absorb that liter of IV fluids in 45 minutes instead of the four hours it will take to drink and absorb that much, it's that 100% of the fluid and anything infused in it is immediately "bioavailable".

If, like at Rapid Recovery, the fluid you receive is Ringer's Lactate (as opposed to "normal saline" which is used in most places and situations), that means you're also receiving calcium chloride, potassium chloride, and both the chloride and lactated forms of sodium, and all are immediately put to use by your body with no lag for absorption time.

More importantly, remember that as you attempt to drink fluids to regain hydration, you're still dehydrated.

Let's assume you ran a 10K in the heat, or worked a double shift, or had food poisoning and are 3 liters of fluid short of optimal hydration. In a study by the University of Montreal, subjects absorbed about half of the 300ml of water they drank in 15 minutes. The other half wasn't fully absorbed for between 75 and 120 minutes. That's a third of a liter. If you're in great shape and absorb an entire liter in two hours, you're still going to be down two liters of fluid after the two hours have passed, and still down a liter after four hours.

For simple dehydration, IV fluid replacement is the most efficient, least cumbersome, best method of rehydration.

2. You're recovering from ILLNESS

We've all had "the crud". Everyone here has had that whopper of a cold that lasted 5 days, strep throat, the flu, or something similar.

It didn't take long, even if you weren't throwing up constantly, to become dehydrated. Lack of fluid intake and sweating profusely will drain your body of fluids in a very short period of time. If you suffered from nausea and vomiting during your illness, the dehydration came more quickly and more dramatically.

You know that your body is a machine that needs all parts working in unison to operate properly. When you're weakened from lack of food intake, fever, and/or dehydration, your immune system can't do its job to properly combat the infection you're fighting, whether it's bacterial or viral.

Unfortunately, the dehydration is not the end of the negative impact on your system. You're missing critical vitamins, minerals, electrolytes and nutrients if you aren't eating properly or drinking water and other fortified fluids.

Things like Vitamin C, Vitamin D, Zinc, Magnesium and Potassium are critical to organ function and immune system health, and you simply aren't getting them when you're sick or recovering from illness if you can't eat and drink normally. There's just not a quick way to receive all the nutrients you need from oral intake.

If you're responsible for cooking in your home and are unable to cook foods that contain what you need, if you're unable to "keep down" foods, or if the person who is responsible finds that they're not capable of getting you to eat the nutrient rich foods that your body needs during illness, you may find yourself in a hole that's deeper than dehydration.

Even if you are able to "keep down" some foods, odds are you're eating quick, processed foods, whether from a restaurant, a delivery service, or something packaged from a store. Foods like shellfish, dark leafy greens, and red meat, which replace the nutrients you've lost, are likely not on your menu, even if you aren't throwing up.

During and after illness not only do you need fluid replacement, you need nutrient replacement. No amount of beef broth is going to get your body back where it needs to be. IV fluids can be infused with a multitude of vitamins, electrolytes, and nutrients.

Urgent care centers and hospital emergency rooms are geared to treat the immediate symptoms and emergent needs of patients, and may not infuse your IV with additives/multivitamins which can help replace some of the critical building blocks you need. IV spas will often offer a wide array of supplemental nutrients that you can have infused, such as Thiamine, Niacin, B12, B-Complex, Zinc, Magnesium, Folic Acid, and others.

When you're simply dehydrated from the lake, the game, the job, or the sun there's no need to specifically request the nutrients we listed above. When you're sick, or when you've been sick and are recovering, you're going to need more than just fluids. You're going to need to replace the nutrients you've lost, and you're going to need them relatively quickly.

IV is unquestionably the better choice for fluid and nutrient replacement for these patients.

3. You have a MIGRAINE, or feel one coming

Got ya didn't we? An IV for a migraine?

Many migraine sufferers have spent years and thousands upon thousands of dollars trying every medication on the market. They've tried Relpax, Imitrex, high dose aspirin, Zomig, Maxalt, and dozens of others.

Some who prefer to stay away from prescription medicine try over the counter remedies like magnesium supplements, fish oil capsules, and ginger root pills.

Many have resorted to herbal and homemade remedies like peppermint oil on their temples, lavender scent diffusers, incense, and frozen headbands.

There is an endless supply of information about migraines and their prevention. We even wrote a migraine resource paper that ended up nearly thirty pages long full of our favorite tips and tricks for avoiding a migraine or stopping one once it has started. You can find it at https://www.rapidrecoveryroom.com/migraine-resource-paper-2019. That's not why we're here though. We're here to discuss whether or not, and if so how, an IV is appropriate for a person suffering from a migraine.

As you know, most headaches, migraines included, involve vasoconstriction. Much of vasoconstriction is caused by dehydration. Immediate hydration can relieve one of the main causes of migraines.

More importantly, as we've already discussed, whatever is infused into your IV bag is immediately put to use by your body. That being the case, there's no waiting for your digestive tract to break down a pain reliever and distribute it appropriately. There's no lengthy wait for the anti-nausea med to work its way through your system. Given properly, with the right additives in the right setting, an IV can be a near instant cure for a migraine.

In most quality IV treatment centers your IV will be administered in a cool, quiet, dark room, and you will most likely find yourself in a cushy recliner. Calming the noise, eliminating the distractions, and making sure that light sensitivity is addressed are all important parts of any rapid response to a migraine.

In general, you'll be administered a liter of fluids with a few important additives. The first of those will be a pain reliever. The greatest probability is that you'll be given Toradol, or its generic equivalent Ketorolac. Your dosage will depend on your weight, kidney function, and how long it has been since you last took a pain reliever, among other things. Ketorolac is an NSAID (Non-Steroidal Anti-Inflammatory Drug). Think of Advil, Aspirin, Anaprox, et al. The goal is to 1) dilate your blood vessels to end the "throbbing" feeling caused by vasoconstriction, and 2) relieve any muscle tension which is likely adding to the tension which causes migraines.

You may also be given Ondansetron (brand name Zofran) to combat nausea. Some IV therapy centers will use Phenergan, but because it has risks that include tissue necrosis if a vein is not properly "hit", it's much less common than Zofran. It also causes drowsiness and it's not safe to have before driving, so again, most IV centers will shy away from Phenergan, but it is used in some places, under certain circumstances. That said, you're probably going to get Ondansetron. It's VERY important to let your provider know if you may be pregnant. Some studies have shown Ondansetron to be linked to an increase in birth defects in the first 12 weeks of pregnancy. In general, at 13 weeks or beyond Ondansetron has shown to be harmless, though some providers will still not offer it to pregnant patients even at that point. Remember, you may not KNOW you're pregnant at 9 or 10 weeks, that's why it's important to remember that the proper question is whether or not you MAY be pregnant.

Nearly all migraine-treatment IVs will include magnesium. Used as an anti-cramping agent, magnesium will likely lower your blood pressure, and reduce whatever muscle spasms, tension, or cramps you may be feeling. Lower blood pressure should immediately help with your "throb". Though muscle tension isn't directly part of the pounding in your head, it can trigger a migraine AND keep you from being able to end one. Not having tight muscles in your neck or shoulders makes it much easier to relax and let the medicine do its work.

Lastly, but importantly, many IV therapy centers will offer medical grade oxygen to their migraine treatment patients. You can expect about a half an hour of oxygen at two liters per minute by nasal cannula. Oxygen is a fantastic vasodilator and will be another arrow in the quiver of things that relieve that thumping pressure. Further, oxygen in your bloodstream helps break down lactic acid, which means you can more easily fight off any muscular tension or spasms.

As with nearly all other migraine treatments, most patients who benefit from IV treatment eventually experience tachyphylaxis, which means that over time treatments become less and less effective. In our center we've seen patients swear by the Migraine Package for a few months, then see it working relatively well but not nearly to the extent it was initially, and eventually by month six or so there's little point in the treatment at all. We have found that taking a break (also about 6 months) can make the treatment more effective when it's restarted. Sadly, in our personal experience this seems to be true of most all migraine treatments, and IV migraine treatment is no different.

4. You're recovering from an ATHLETIC event

Sports drinks are great… for your kids… after school.

A typical 16 oz. sports drink contains 34 grams of sugar. That's about 15% of your entire average daily requirement. It also has about 270mg of basic table salt. Not kosher sea salt,

Himalayan pink salt, or anything with any kind of additional mineral content or benefits, plain old white table salt, and about 15% of your required daily intake.

That's essentially it. Most contain between 2 and 5 percent of your daily dose of potassium, and some contain a little citric acid, which you probably know comes from citrus fruits like oranges, lemons, or grapefruits. Despite the fact that some do contain citric acid, there's not enough to amount to anything more than the ability of the maker to put "contains real fruit juice" on the label.

They aren't going to "get you back in the game" or "help you recover" appreciably faster or better than tap water.

"But wait," you say, "those drinks are loaded with electrolytes." Well, yes and no. Without getting into the science of electrolytic function, salt and potassium are the "electrolytes" you're getting from a sports drink. Very little potassium at that. You're just as well off with a banana and a glass of water.

Let's say your team won the first two games in a softball tournament and you played in the 9:30 championship. Maybe you had a tennis tournament at your club. You finished 18 holes and when you were in the clubhouse someone talked you into another round. Your workout went longer than expected.

You're dehydrated. You've got some leg cramps. You sweated out Lord knows what amount of electrolytes. Because you spent the entire day being active there's a pretty good chance you didn't eat right.

You're suffering from muscle strain, soreness, dehydration, and possibly secondary effects like muscle cramps and headache.

The first thing your body needs is the fluids. That's a given.

You've heard your body needs more. Gatorade tells you that every time you turn on the television. If you need "more" the IV will give it to you.

In general, athletic recovery IVs will contain a mix of minerals like magnesium to calm muscle spasms, amino acids to speed recovery, and most likely some type of med for the soreness. At Rapid Recovery the "Game Changer" contains meds, minerals, vitamins, and OAC (Ornithine, Arginine, and Citrulline), to improve blood flow, increase metabolism, and speed recovery. Most of the additives in athletic recovery IVs can be taken BEFORE athletic activities to improve performance, but are well suited to muscle repair and relief after strenuous exercise or activity.

Gatorade is developing a patch to determine exactly what you've sweated out of your body and will ultimately tailor a drink to your losses, but until that happens, IV is the vastly superior option.

5. You got FOOD POISONING

This is one of the most common reasons people seek IV treatment in and out of urgent care settings.

Let's start at the beginning. Day One. You threw up whatever you ate. You stayed in the bathroom and vomited repeatedly. That's awful for your body. You lost a TON of fluids. Whatever nutrition you consumed you didn't absorb. Your muscles are racked with pain from the heaving. If you're lucky you didn't end up with diarrhea. If you weren't lucky, you lost even more fluid.

Day Two rolls around and you're weak and dehydrated. You aren't throwing up repeatedly, but if you eat anything or drink more than enough to keep your mouth moist, you throw up again. So, since that's no fun you don't drink anything.

You need SEVERAL things. 1) You need fluids. 2) You need something to calm the spasms in your stomach. 3) You need something to stop the vomiting immediately. 4) You need something for the muscle pain. 5) You need to replace the nutrients you haven't absorbed.

It's all bad, but you are the classic candidate to get IV therapy at an IV treatment spa and see a big turnaround quickly.

You look like hell. It's okay. You've been sick. You don't want to put on your jammies and head to Quick Care. Put on your jammies and head to an IV treatment center. I promise you aren't the first, and you won't be the last. Everyone there, doctors, nurses, staff, and other patients, knows exactly what you're going through. Someone kind will put you in a private room and you can fall asleep immediately, in your fat pants and a sweatshirt.

Once you're there you're going to get something in your IV to calm/sooth your stomach. You're probably still having cramping and a sour feel in your belly. Odds are you'll be infused with a medicine called Famotidine.

This is where you have to be honest with your IV center. Famotidine has some interactions with ibuprofen, and also interacts with acetaminophen. You'll want to let your IV specialist know if you've taken either of those meds so they can decide whether or not you should receive Famotidine.

If you're in great heart health you may also get Ondansetron (Zofran), though there is a rarely occurring interaction between the two drugs that can cause an irregular heart rhythm that can be dangerous.

If you're worried that because you've been nauseated you might find yourself throwing up in the IV center, don't. As we said before, you aren't the first and you won't be the last. Most IV centers actually have a big box of things called "emesis bags", which is what the rest of us call "barf bags". The doctors, nurses, and/or paramedics you're dealing with (depending on which center is providing your treatment) have seen nausea and anything else you can throw at them more times than you can count. It won't bother them a bit.

6. You're "worn down"

"I'm worn down" is a very common phrase in phone calls to IV centers. "I just don't feel right", "I guess I haven't been eating well", "I'm just 'off' since my vacation", and "I'm working all the time and I'm trying to keep the house together and I'm about to collapse" get told to IV centers time after time after time.

You're a mother. You get up at 6:30 to take your teenage daughter to school. Since she hasn't quite mastered the art of doing everything she's supposed to do to be waiting at the car with a smile, you have to get up a half an hour early to help her along.

Then you head to work. Half the people there know you're the "go-to" person when something is important, so your work area looks like a tornado blew through it. You get something awful for lunch, but quick, and get right back at the grind.

Whoops. You aren't drinking enough water, but we'll get to that later. You work past 5, and fight traffic on the way home.

Hey, congratulations, there's only about 10 minutes worth of cleaning up other people's stuff before you start cooking dinner, or maybe you just order something not-so-good-for-you.

The good news is that there's enough time to get two loads of laundry done before you go to bed and get ready to do it all again tomorrow.

How long can you keep that up without wearing down to the point that your immune system is shot, you have bags under your eyes, you're wrinkled from dehydration, your body starts performing poorly due to lack of proper nutrition, and you feel like you're going to collapse?

Not long. You can go get a massage, or spend a day at the pool, or just take a day off, but none of those things will replace the nutrients you haven't been getting or the fluids you're lacking.

No IV center or bar or spa can "cure" the problem you're having with running yourself ragged, but they can jumpstart the process. You're going to have to start taking care of yourself, but getting fluids, some Vitamin C, some B12, magnesium to work down that tension in your neck, a little folic acid, and thiamine will go a long way toward at least getting you back into some kind of balance. You'll pass some of it in your urine because you won't be completely deficient in all of those vitamins, but you'll surely be "topped off" so to speak.

7. "One last round" got ordered 4 times

It happens. You have a glass of wine waiting to be seated for dinner, then you have another with dinner. You aren't driving so you have one more with dessert. On your way out you see Mark and Terri and they're going to a little pub next door to the restaurant. Why not?

The next thing you know the sun is peeking through the shutters, your head is pounding, the bathroom door is still open, your socks are on the floor in front of the toilet, and you realize you've got to take your kid to an 11 a.m. soccer game.

At this point you're thinking you can take a few Advil, drink a half a bottle of Pedialyte, maybe eat a banana, get 30 more minutes of sleep and work your way through it.

We've all done it. Let's face it, even with that plan, it sucks. Worse, you may be doing yourself more harm than good. Pain relievers like Advil and Anaprox (naproxen sodium) are NSAIDs (non-steroidal anti-inflammatory drugs) which work through your liver, and they're hard on it. Acetaminophen (Tylenol) is a liver-crushing disaster. Most of these pain relievers are fine if you've taken in enough fluids to process them safely, but half the reason you're hung over is that you're dehydrated, and you simply can't drink enough fluids in a short period of time to make them as safe as they should be.

So first let's explore what is happening inside your body, and what needs to be fixed, then we'll talk about how an IV is the best bet for doing just that.

First, no matter how much liquid you put into your system last night, you're dehydrated. Two reasons: 1) Alcohol isn't water. There's no hydration value in it. Though it's a liquid, it actually serves to dehydrate you. 2) Alcohol inhibits the release of a hormone called vasopressin, which limits your body's urine output. You likely went to the restroom more than you remember. That serves to dehydrate you more than you otherwise would be.

Second, you might not realize it, but you likely sweated quite a bit. Sadly, it was probably when you were throwing up. Both of those things serve to really dehydrate you.

So what? You're dehydrated. What's the big deal? Well, dehydration causes something called vasoconstriction. That's what gives you the throbbing headache. Pain reliever can help, but if you want to fight vasoconstriction you need fluids in a hurry. You just can't absorb enough water or Gatorade in a quick enough time period for it to be effective. Pedialyte? Sure. I've done it. It's better than water or a sports drink, but it's not playing the same game as balanced fluids full of electrolytes sent directly into your bloodstream. If drinking water is a 1 on a scale of 1 to 10, Gatorade is a 2 and Pedialyte is a 4. You need a 10. IV fluids are a 10.

Fluids are going to help, but they aren't going to complete the job. You're still minus a LOT of critical vitamins and minerals. Most "retail" IV centers load up plenty of good vitamins and minerals in their "hangover cure" IV bags. You can almost be certain you'll receive a fairly high dose of B vitamins. Your body burns through B when you're drinking/hungover, and it's a big deal to have it replaced immediately via IV.

Potassium is another hugely important additive that most places have in their hangover cures. It can come in the form of lactated potassium in Ringer's Lactate, be in a multi-vitamin that's added to your bag, or can be infused as a stand-alone additive (rare, but does happen). Potassium helps keep you from having a thready heartbeat, and can relieve muscle cramps. When oxygenated blood isn't pumping steadily you face two symptoms: an uneasy, "uncentered" feeling, and a build-up of lactic acid in your muscles. The whole thing leads to that shakiness you have during a hangover. The potassium is key to relieving those symptoms.

Other common additives are magnesium for muscle cramps, thiamine, folic acid, and a broad-spectrum multi-vitamin. Most are included simply to replace what you've burned off or thrown up, though the magnesium is specifically used as a muscle relaxant to relieve cramping and muscle tightness/soreness.

Many IV centers today will also treat you with 2 liters per minute of pure oxygen via nasal cannula. Though you likely don't "need" oxygen the way a COPD patient would, it causes vasodilation and greatly reduces headache, throbbing, and the "brain fog" you experience as a result of constricted veins and higher blood pressure (required to move consistent amounts of oxygenated blood).

8. Immunity Boost for Wellness Care

Before we go into the benefits of an IV packed with immune boosting goodies, let's clear up something immediately: NOTHING can replace a healthy diet (rich in fruits, vegetables, and lean meats), fresh air and sunshine, consistent hydration, and plenty of quality sleep, when it comes to supporting your immune system.

That said, we all fall short of optimal nutrition, hydration, and sleep occasionally.

Most "Immune Booster" IVs contain a LOT of Vitamin C. Honestly, most are probably overdone with C. It's one thing to give someone 3 to 5 grams, but you'll find as much as 15 grams of Vitamin C in many IV centers' immunity booster IVs. That's pointless. There's a very good chance anything above 5g is simply going to end up in your toilet after you've urinated. Five grams might as well, but that's really the high end of what you need to get the anti-inflammatory effects, and other immune benefits.

At our IV center we include zinc, as do most other similar centers, but it's less for boosting your immune system than it is for shortening the length of a cold or other virus. The exact mechanism isn't fully understood, but clinical studies have shown that high amounts of zinc tend to shorten the length of a cold by as much as a day or two. It's more of a "can't hurt" addition to an immune program IV.

Just as common in these treatments is a strong antioxidant called glutathione. Antioxidants remove free radicals, preventing cellular damage. Stronger cells are far less likely to succumb to viruses. Though you aren't particularly "boosting" your immune system by revving up your antioxidant intake, you're giving the rest of your body a better chance at fighting off an infection.

No quality immunity booster IV therapy is complete without a solid multi-vitamin. Why? Any deficiency gives a virus a crack in the armor to attack you. Most good multi-vitamins contain Vitamin D, several B vitamins, C, E, K, and trace elements. Though your body may not need ALL of those vitamins, a broad spectrum vitamin covers all the bases without expensive lab work. You're likely to urinate out most of it, but it's that one little thing you're lacking that might make the difference, and a broad spectrum multi-vitamin will cover that gap.

You still have to wash your hands. You still can't drink after people. There's still no such thing as the "5 second rule". No "Immune Boost IV" is going to make you impervious to infection, but it's a good start, especially when nastiness is going around and your system isn't up to the task by itself.

9. You're trying to "max out" your game

This one is tricky. Not because it's hard to decide what you want, but because there's not nearly as much evidence of efficacy (effectiveness) for most of these types of treatments.

You'll see these treatments advertised everywhere. They say things like "rock your workout", "live your best life", or "accelerate your game". If you see anything like that, read it all twice, ask a bunch of questions, and be skeptical.

Some are based in science, some in schlock.

If you're an athlete you can reliably expect some results from the IV treatments that contain, or are followed by injections of, various amino acids. Many contain some form or other of Arginine, Citrulline, Ornithine, Lysine, and others. The majority of those aminos are intended to do one thing: increase oxygen to your muscles through one mechanism or another. They either increase your blood flow, the ability of your red blood cells to carry oxygen molecules, or carry on some other function intended to let your body "grow" (that doesn't really happen but it's a good basic explanation) muscle, or repair muscle damage quickly.

One or two of these treatments probably isn't going to help much unless you've overdone it and are looking for a quicker rebound. If you're trying to build muscle, get to a personal record, or really tear into your competition you need to be on a regular routine of these types of aminos.

There are two big problems with these types of treatments. The first is that there hasn't been a lot of high-quality, non-sponsored scientific study regarding the long-term use of these supplements and their effects on the body. We just don't know. Now, you're going to find some guy in a local gym whose arms are bigger around than your thighs and he's going to tell you about all the aminos he pounds like water, but it's probably a good idea to check back with him in a few years and find out if he still has a liver, or if he's had a stroke. We offer these at our spa, but we're pretty cautious about them.

The next big problem is that if you're REALLY into some kind of serious competitive situation, there's a good chance your governing body prohibits them. We've had hockey organizations, the PGA, MMA, the USTA, and other professional leagues, as well as some colleges, tell us that their athletes will be guilty of taking performance enhancing drugs if they have elevated levels of some of these aminos in their blood.

10. Mental clarity/support

Several years ago a large, well-run study showed some amazing results. Mice with mental and memory impairment (similar to Parkinson's or dementia) were given NAD+ (nicotinamide adenine dinucleotide), and a pretty shocking number of them not only showed a halt in the progression of the malady as compared to the mice not given NAD+, many showed a reversal of their symptoms.

Put simply, Nicotinamide Adenine Dinucleotide (NAD+) is a "cofactor" in cellular metabolism. A "cofactor" is a molecule (chemical compound) necessary for an enzyme to function. It's called a "dinucleotide" because it's a group of two nucleotides (one is nicotinamide and the other is an adenine nucleobase) which are joined together by a phosphate group. You can think of it as a double railcar joined together with a link, that moves material from one station to another to allow the work at the receiving station to progress.

The simplest way to put what NAD+ is/does is that it moves electrons from Point A to Point B, so the station at Point B can use the electrons to perform a job. NAD+ "picks up" a Hydrogen molecule (one electron), becomes NADH, then essentially deposits the electron and becomes NAD+ again. The electron is now in the mitochondria (remember your teacher calling it the "power plant of the cell"?), helps generate ATP, and the product created is used to power the specific function of the cell.

So, why does it matter? Well, imagine your memory as a computer chip running at 60% power. Now imagine you introduce something to increase the transfer of electricity from the outlet to the computer chip. Viola. More computing power. Think of a cell that's in the process of undergoing repair. More fuel to repair means a quicker, more efficient repair job. Anything a cell does in your body can be done better by that cell if it has a quicker, larger energy supply.

Now you're wondering what people claim it's good for, and what kind of proof there is.

Probably the best studied use for NAD+ is improved cognition. The massive study of mice showed that those with signs of cognitive impairment improved fairly dramatically with large, frequent doses of NAD. Remember, that's just mice, but brain functions are very similar in most mammals, suggesting improved cognition in humans who use NAD is likely. Many physicians use NAD infusions or injections to fight the effects of Parkinson's and Alzheimer's. A complete, double-blind, controlled study hasn't been conducted in enough humans to determine if people without any mental impairment benefit from NAD to the extent of increased mental capacity/function, but it's certainly a logical conclusion that they would.

WebMD says "NAD(H) is used for improving mental clarity, alertness, concentration, and memory; as well as for treating Alzheimer's disease and dementia." They do go on to say that there isn't sufficient testing to prove that it works effectively, but until there are prolonged, placebo controlled, double-blind studies in large groups of humans, we won't have all the data we need.

NAD+ has been shown in clinical studies to improve liver function and repair liver damage in mice. Mice again... but that's where all clinical trials start.

Other than focus, the most common use for NAD is to combat chronic fatigue. WebMD (again) does say that NAD has shown effectiveness in fighting the symptoms of chronic fatigue, which makes sense as NAD is used by your mitochondria to increase metabolic rates in cells. Athletes worldwide have been using NAD infusions and supplements to enhance performance, though many sports governing bodies have added NAD to their "performance enhancing drug" list, prohibiting its use in many sanctioned events and leagues.

Here's the one you're all waiting to hear: Does NAD extend your lifespan? You can't really expect us to say "of course it does". Here's what had led to that claim: In 2013 a study was published in Neurobiology of Aging that had results which suggested that the deterioration of cognition was slowed significantly, if not reversed, in mice which were given increased levels of NAD. That's not to say that a 60 year old suddenly stops aging, but that the decline of the cells tested almost entirely halted. Now those mice were given a boatload of NAD, and they certainly weren't checked for other possible long-term side-effects, but the data did suggest that the expected age-related deterioration of the studied cells halted. You make of that what you will. We wouldn't claim anything other than that we read the study and it excited us too.

So, what is it? Uncle Sham's Miracle Elixir of Complete BS, or super supplement? We can't say. There aren't enough tests, but there's no question that many people who use NAD regularly swear by it. It certainly has an immediate, recognizable physical effect on your body, suggesting at least some efficacy.

11. You're Receiving Chemotherapy

Can you say "sucks" in a book? We vote yes. So, not only does cancer suck, chemotherapy sucks. You already know this by now, but you're essentially poisoning yourself to kill the cancer cells. Though chemotherapy has come a long way, areas can be targeted, and your chemo team can try to limit the damage to the rest of your body, poison is poison.

So you sit in an infusion center chair, get a bunch of chemo, and the next day you're beaten up like you've been in a fight, you're nauseated, you have a headache, and you just feel miserable. You probably aren't eating a whole bunch either. Really all you want to do is sleep and wake up when you feel more like yourself.

Most IV centers see lots of chemo patients. They know what you're going through, and what it takes to help.

You'll get a liter of fluids from most places, though getting two liters isn't uncommon. What you need to pay attention to is what goes in the fluids, and whether or not the center can customize your treatment.

For starters, you're absolutely going to need an anti-nausea med. Some cities use Phenergan, which is incredibly effective but has drawbacks. If a vein isn't properly "hit", Phenergan can cause tissue necrosis. You absolutely do not want that, because it's just what it says it is, dying tissue. YOUR tissue. It's pretty rare, but if a nurse misses you could be in some trouble with Phenergan. Just as importantly, you're either going to have to have a ride home or take a ride service, because Phenergan causes drowsiness, and you are definitely not supposed to drive after getting it. For those reasons most places use Zofran, or its generic form called Ondansetron. Zofran isn't quite as effective as Phenergan, but it's plenty good for what you (or your loved one) will need, and most IV centers consider it safer.

You're also going to need some kind of pain reliever. Almost every IV center uses Ketorolac, which you may know as

Toradol. Basically you're getting instantly effective, high-potency NSAID for pain.

Some places don't tend to put in much more than a B-complex, and that's a mistake. The B-complex is great for an energy boost. You want that. You might get Thiamine and Folic Acid as well. Great. Those are excellent B-vitamins. They aren't enough. The problem is, chemo patients feel like hell and tend not to eat much, and if they do they aren't eating a good balanced diet. You (or they) need a full-spectrum multi-vitamin. Make sure what you're getting has A, D, E, and a nice solid balance.

Here's something to be aware of: Vitamin C might not be your best idea after chemo. Yes, it's a great thing 99 times out of 100, but this isn't the time you want an anti-inflammatory. You're already dehydrated, and odds are what's causing your body grief has nothing to do with inflammation. Plenty of people think Vitamin C is some kind of miracle cancer cure (which we discussed earlier), but after getting chemo, loading up on an anti-inflammatory doesn't feel like it makes much sense.

Of all the times you want to be able to get exactly what you want, and nothing you don't, post-chemo IV therapy is the big one. If your nearest IV center gets their treatments pre-prepared from some mail order corporate center, keep driving and find the closest one that mixes its own.

12. Jet Lag

The gist of jet lag boils down to dehydration, and the physical "drag" of being low on energy due to a time change. You can easily spend two days "normalizing" your body after a long flight, most especially when you left somewhere at noon, your body is planning to be in bed in 11 hours, but instead of 11 hours later being 11 o'clock at night, it's only 7 o'clock and you have obligations.

Most of the jet lag IVs you'll see are absolutely crammed with various kinds of Vitamin B. The fluids are obviously to rehydrate you, and the B vitamins give you the energy you need to make it through those extra hours so you can get your body's rhythm back on track.

It's not a magic trick. It's pretty simple. Replace what you lost, and give you a little extra boost of energy to get through until you can go to sleep tonight, and wake up tomorrow on a normal schedule.

13. Elevation sickness

The concentration of oxygen in the air is the same at 20,000 feet as it is at 2,000 feet. The problem is the lack of atmospheric pressure. Think of it like this: Two parts of Koolaid in 8 parts water is exactly the same ratio in a gallon as it is in a thimble. At lower altitudes you're getting a gallon. In Denver, you're trying to breathe a thimbleful of air at 5,500 feet (at least compared to sea level), and that causes problems.

Worse, because of the lack of moisture in the air you're rapidly becoming dehydrated, as your lungs outgas water vapor into the drier air. In the South we're used to sticky humidity. Up in the mountains, snow or not, the air is dry as a bone. So, you're breathing out moisture with every breath.

The common elevation sickness IV contains some of the same amino acids that you'll find in athletic recovery IVs. The trick to those aminos is their ability to help your tissues (muscles) absorb oxygen. Decreased oxygen saturation is your biggest problem and those aminos are included specifically to eliminate that problem. All of them, ornithine, arginine, et al, are aminos that specifically help transport oxygen into your tissues.

You'll also get an NSAID pain reliever to help with the headache. The headache is caused by vasoconstriction, and lower oxygen levels in your brain, and the NSAID will help knock that out while the aminos do their work, and your body acclimatizes to the altitude.

One of these treatments may not be enough, depending on the change in altitude you've experienced. Typically you should only add about 1,000 to 1,500 feet of altitude a day to avoid the effects of elevation sickness, and shouldn't expect to fully acclimatize to heights above 5,500 feet for at least a few days. The problem, obviously, is that you leave Houston at noon, and by 4 you're in Aspen and you've picked up 6,000 feet in 4 hours. Hence, the whole "elevation sickness" IV craze.

Don't be surprised if you're at Elevation Hydration in Colorado Springs on the first day of your ski trip, getting your nausea, shortness of breath, and headache fixed, and see a bunch of other lowlands people sitting next to you.

CHAPTER 2:

So, Why an IV Instead of Oral Fluids and Supplements?

If you're reading this book, you likely know the answer, and it's a simple one: Immediate bioavailability.

It boils down to this: Most of what you take in orally is a waste. Your body doesn't process it through your kidneys, and you pass it through your urine. You take 100 milligrams of something, and if everything is just right you absorb maybe 50% of it. The rest ends up in your town's wastewater treatment plant.

Why not just take one of those "Vitamin a Day" gummies you can buy in the store, or a supplement, with food? Ever wonder why with food? For one thing, they upset your stomach because they're massive doses of vitamins and minerals so they can make sure you get some of what you want. Wait, what? Yes. Studies show that only just more than half of what you swallow makes it into your bloodstream, even if you've got the dead right pill and take it at the dead right time(*). Secondly, the acid in your stomach that's churning when you eat helps break down the pills and allows some of the wanted ingredient to get into the blood stream

Sometimes the pills don't break down effectively and you absorb about 3% of the actual vitamin or supplement you've taken.

There are far too many vitamins, meds, and supplements, and associated consumption factors, to paint all oral absorption with a broad brush, but suffice it to say you're swallowing it but there's a good chance you aren't absorbing it.

It probably seems obvious because it's going straight into your bloodstream, but nearly 100% of the vitamin/supplement you're receiving through your IV is being absorbed by your body(**). There's a study out there that says only 98% of IV vitamins are absorbed. "Just" 98%. Still beats 3%... or even 50.

And that goes for...

meds, electrolytes, and aminos too. Putting something directly into your bloodstream provides much quicker, much more efficient delivery to your body than swallowing it into your stomach and expecting it to work its way through your GI tract.

* National Institutes of Health (part of the Department of Health and Human Services) study discussing the absorption of oral vitamins. (https://www.ncbi.nlm.nih.gov/pubmed/23989008)

** World Health Organization (W.H.O.) research (http://www.who.int/occupational_health/activities/5injvsora.pdf) showing IV nutrients "nearly 100% bioavailable" versus poor nutrient absorption if taken orally.

Just as importantly, in order to absorb a liter of fluids and have it usable by your system, you really need to drink about a gallon of water. Do you want to drink a gallon of water in an hour?

CHAPTER 3:

Why Shouldn't You Get an IV?

1. You Want to Cure Your _____

A lot of people are under the mistaken impression that whatever ailment they're experiencing can be fixed by SOME IV, if they just find the right one.

Sadly, that's not the case. Some things require more than you can get in a bag of fluids.

An IV can "cure" a hangover. It can "cure" dehydration. It can "cure" a migraine. Those are about it though.

Many people will go to an IV center/bar/spa because they feel "run down", as we've discussed before. Maybe they get a multi-vitamin, or a B12 injection, and they expect that they're going to be "cured". It can happen. Maybe they were just dehydrated. Maybe they were lacking potassium or niacin and just needed to get back "on kilter".

That said, sometimes you get the IV and that's just not enough. So, a week later you're back for another IV. Two weeks after that you change up what you have added to your IV, but you're getting another and hoping that whatever the new additive is will get you back up to snuff.

At this point, if you've tried a few different packages and you're still not feeling right, that IV center isn't going to be your answer.

You know what's coming next: Nothing beats a trip to your primary care provider. They can run a complete blood count, a full lab panel, and many other tests. Maybe you have sleep apnea and don't realize it. You might fall asleep at 11, get up at 7, and not have had a full hour of REM sleep. You can get an IV every day and it isn't going to fix that.

You're just going to have to bite the bullet and see a doctor. We've sent plenty of people to theirs, or one we recommend. That doesn't mean the doctor won't say "oh look, your tests came back and you need to do x, y, and z, and yeah, that multi-vitamin IV every other week is a good idea also", but some things require more than an IV center can do.

Remember, there's a very good reason almost every reputable IV center has a disclaimer at the bottom of every one of the pages on their website that reads something like "The services provided have not been evaluated by the Food and Drug Administration. These products are not intended to diagnose, treat, cure or prevent any disease. The material on this website is provided for informational purposes only and is not medical advice. Always consult your physician before beginning any therapy program. References to therapies are for marketing purposes only and do not guarantee results." Any IV center that guarantees you results for anything other than rehydrating you, or maybe curing a hangover, is simply full of crap. Most of us genuinely believe we can help, but until and unless there are large-scale, double-blind, controlled tests versus placebos for a wide variety of IV therapies, guarantees are dangerous and probably illegal.

2. You're Trying to Overcome Complications From Drug Use

This will be a quick section. You're wasting your time.

Yes, a lot of people who decide to do something stupid find themselves in a bad way, and some percentage of them try to roll into an IV center to get something infused that will help get their body back to normal.

There's nothing at your local IV spa that's going to set your body or your mind right after cocaine, methamphetamine, Xanax, or anything similar. Nobody puts Narcan in an IV. I have seen one or two places nationally that offer something like this, but they're sketchy at best and you're simply better off heading to the ER.

If you know someone who is in a bad way because they did a bunch of drugs, or if you did them yourself, PLEASE do not show up at an IV center. Not only can they not help anyone who's under the influence of a controlled substance, they're going to be put in a really bad position.

A person who is suffering ill effects from drug use needs to be in an emergency room. Yeah, they'll get in some trouble, but they'll probably live, and that's got to be the first priority.

3. You Want to "Detox" For a Drug Test

Also, not gonna happen. Nobody of whom we're aware gives anything in an IV that masks drug use.

Does the fluid help "flush you out"? Probably, but those tests are pretty sophisticated and can tell that you've overloaded on fluids to flush out your system.

So that's really the short answer. No reputable place, even if they offer a "cleanse" package, offers a way to help you beat a drug test. The "cleanse" they're referring to means flushing your system of a wide array of toxins, and is meant to get you back to some sort of balance, not remove all trace of drug use. There's an old saying "the solution to pollution is dilution," but that's more about drinking water when drinking alcohol than it is about getting past a toxicology screen.

If you've made the ill-advised decision to do something that's going to keep you from passing a drug test, your best bet is to buy one of those drinks you find at what we used to call a "head shop", or buy something off the internet. Someone might sell you an IV that they think might help, and you might pay a bunch and cross your fingers, but it's not going to help and you're going to have spent a lot of money and lost your job anyway.

4. You Have Purchased Something You Want Infused

If you bought something on the internet, or from someone you know, or from Canada, or even from a local pharmacy, and an IV center is willing to put it in an IV for you, you better run like hell.

There's absolutely no way for them to know if you've stored it properly, if it's what it says it is, or if it's properly prescribed. They're absolutely risking their medical licenses, their livelihoods, and your life.

I can't stress this enough: If they're willing to break the law to make a dollar by giving you something they can't verify and haven't purchased themselves, they're willing to cut other corners as well. You're in pretty clear danger if you deal with someone like this.

5. You're Pregnant and Have Morning Sickness

This is a controversial one. Some places around the country will give IVs to pregnant women, and some won't.

Four out of 5 pregnant women suffer morning sickness. I know it's a miserable way to start your day, and you'd love some help. You'll end up with sore shoulders, neck pain, and you're dehydrated.

An IV with a little pain reliever and anti-nausea med sounds like a fantastic idea. The problem is that anything you get, your baby gets too.

There are studies that show that Zofran can cause birth defects, especially before you're 13 weeks pregnant. There are studies that show it doesn't. It's pretty commonly accepted among Obstetricians that once the pregnancy gets to 13 weeks Zofran in small amounts can be safely administered to pregnant women. At our IV spas we still don't do it. We're just very, very cautious about pregnancy. Some will do it, though. A phone call will usually get you the answer you need, and most places (if they don't treat pregnant women) will at the very least refer you to someone who does.

Another issue during pregnancy is elevated blood pressure. Some additives commonly used in IVs, and even the increased fluid levels associated with receiving an IV, can increase your blood pressure. The last thing you want when pregnant is a BP spike.

Your best bet is to ASK YOUR OBSTETRICIAN. I can't be more plain or serious about that. Nobody knows your pregnancy (and the implications of procedures on it) better than your Obstetrician. Matter of fact, at our IV centers we only treat pregnant woman with a note from their treating OB, and even then only with simple fluids. That causes us a lot of grief and upsets a lot of people, but pregnancy is serious business, and the OB ALWAYS knows best.

6. You're Trying to Get Treatment for a Minor

As with pregnancy, there are exceptions to the "no minors" policy most IV centers have. Some will treat minors under certain circumstances.

Remember, minors' bodies haven't fully developed. They haven't encountered enough different things for anyone to have a complete grasp on their allergies. They may have blood pressure spikes. There are just more variables and more risks to giving a minor an IV than there are to giving a healthy adult an IV.

Some centers will, if a parent or guardian is present, treat more physically mature minors if there is a Parental Consent form signed. There's still usually an age limit and a size limit, commonly 13 or 14 years old, and at least 100 pounds. Most will not however add many of the common additives that may cause an allergic reaction.

At our center we will treat minors if we have both a parental consent AND a note from the child's pediatrician. We also provide pro-bono treatments to pediatric chemotherapy patients if their parent or guardian is present, signs a consent, and the child's treating oncologist or pediatrician authorizes it. Your nearby center may not provide a free treatment, but it's worth explaining the situation if your child is receiving chemo and you need help.

7. You Think You Can Get an IV That Will Cause Weight Loss

You've seen them. They're called "Slim and Trim", "Fat Blaster", "Calorie Burner", and "Belly Buster". They all claim to help you lose weight, and they all cost a fortune.

If you'll pardon the language, they're also all bullshit. Think about it. If you could get an IV that shed your belly fat, you'd never see a single person who had two nickels to rub together who was a single pound overweight.

As close as you could POSSIBLY come to claiming an IV can help you to lose weight is that IF you decided not to eat, and you got all the nutrients your body needs via IV, and therefore burned more calories than you absorbed, you'd lose weight. You could do that with water, supplements, and a strict diet just as easily.

There's a VERY simple formula to lose weight: Burn more calories than you consume. That's it.

The most convincing study we've seen for one of these treatments (an injection called Lipo-B) was a big double-blind controlled study of something like 6,000 people. Half of them ate what was given to them, exercised according to a plan, and took shots of this medication. The other half ate the same thing, exercised according to the same plan, and got a placebo.

The people who got the weight-loss drug lost a little more than 3 pounds more over the course of 6 months than the people who got the placebo. THREE POUNDS. Over 6 months. We charge 40 bucks for those shots (and tell people EXACTLY what we think of them), and the people in the study got them once a week. That's twenty-four $40 shots to lose three pounds. If you do that you'll pay $960 to lose an extra three pounds. You could buy a five dollar bottle of laxative and lose just as much weight (temporarily). Might as well just starve yourself for two days.

If there were an IV that helped people lose weight I'd have so much money I'd be on a beach in Fiji writing this book… and I'm not.

8. You simply can't get your "pep" back.

There are a million reasons you might feel "draggy". Lots of them (improper nutrition, dehydration, low levels of some vitamins, aminos, or trace elements) CAN be fixed with an IV. You might be deficient in Vitamin B, or D, or potassium, and a power-packed IV can help that. Being dehydrated really drags you down. OBVIOULSY an IV can help that.

But let's assume you've been eating right, drinking the appropriate amount of water every day (your body weight in pounds, divided by two, in ounces), haven't been sick, and get 8 hours of sleep a night. What then? Well, there are a bunch of possibilities.

First, you may not be getting "good" sleep. You might have sleep apnea. You might consider an at-home sleep study for a hundred bucks. That's a cheap way to find out if poor sleep is what's bringing you down.

Second, you may have a hormonal issue or some problem with your endocrine system. Maybe you have hypothyroidism. It's not going to be cheap, but a visit to an endocrinologist couldn't hurt. What if they find the one thing your body isn't producing something properly, put you on a med for it (like Synthroid), and you're suddenly Batman? Wouldn't that be worth the money?

What if you aren't absorbing Vitamin D the way you should, and your serum D level is way low? Maybe inexpensive routine Vitamin D shots are the answer.

Hell, it could even be something in your intestinal tract, where you aren't absorbing nutrition the way you should.

What we're saying is, if you try an IV, or two, or three, and you're still feeling draggy, you need more medical help than you can get in a recliner.

9. You Have a Continual Stomach/Gastrointestinal Issue

We see this issue a lot.

So, everyone has eaten something they regretted after the fact. It happened to me just this past Wednesday. I was fairly certain death was next. Today I feel like a champ.

Do you know what that tells me? It was an isolated incident, not indicative of a problem.

If you have bad bathroom issues one day, take some Nauzene or Pepto, and get better, but the same problem comes back in a week, you might have a serious problem.

Most IV centers have a GI package that knocks out just about anything your GI tract can throw at you. That said, if you go in for a GI package on Sunday because you have a stomach problem, and then you're back in a week with the same problem, you might not need an IV, you might need a doctor's appointment.

You could have a GI bleed, excess production of stomach acid, a bacterial infection in your gastrointestinal tract, or even cancer. Unless you're eating at the same dirty street taco stand and get a virus three times in three weeks, getting an IV package for stomach/GI issues ought to be a "once in a blue moon" kind of event.

If a reputable IV center sees you twice in a relatively short period of time they're going to (1) tell you to stop eating wherever you're eating, and/or (2) tell you to schedule a visit with your PCP.

CHAPTER 4:

What You Can Expect to Get at an IV Center

Honestly, you probably aren't even really sure what is in the IV you're being given at most IV centers. We see a lot of IV places around the country that have the EXACT same description of every package they give, with one little change. They'll say something like "a blend of vitamins, electrolytes, and amino acids specifically blended to _____" where the "_____" is what you're trying to accomplish, like "beat a hangover", "help you shed pounds", or "give you a little extra mojo".

You should be concerned if they won't tell you, or God forbid don't know, exactly what is in every package, and why it's in there.

Read and ask. Here are some of the common fluids and additives given at IV centers around the country.

Sodium Chloride: Just like it sounds. Salt water. .9% NACL in water. Many centers use this common, and inexpensive fluid.

Ringer's Lactate: Some centers, in our opinion the better centers, start with a base of 1L of Ringer's Lactate (also called a "balanced bag"), which contains: Calcium chloride, Potassium chloride, Sodium chloride, and Sodium lactate.

Ringer's is more isotonically similar to blood, and has a better mix of electrolytes (salts).

Multi-vitamin: Most centers offer some form of multi-vitamin. Ask about what's in it. Many are just B-complex mixes without much else. Some will also contain a little Vitamin C.

Our multi-vitamin (**Infuvite** by Baxter) contains: Vitamin C, Vitamin A, Vitamin D3, Vitamin B1, Vitamin B2, Vitamin B6, Vitamin B3, Dexpanthenol (a B vitamin), Vitamin E, Vitamin K1, Biotin, Folic Acid, and Vitamin B12.

Thiamine: Also known as B1. Though in most multi-vitamins in small amounts, in some centers you will get extra B1.

Magnesium: Known to ease muscle cramps and tightness, magnesium is essential for proper function of the heart, nerves, and muscles, in addition to being important to cells and bones.

Vitamin C: Critical to your immune system and ability to fight off colds and the flu.

Folic Acid: Also known as B9, folic acid is an essential vitamin which the body uses for cellular division and to combat anemia. Folate deficiency occurs with age, and can be combated by a diet rich in green leafy vegetables. Critical to good health.

Glutathione: A powerful anti-oxidant, glutathione is thought to promote cellular health by preventing damage due to free radicals, peroxides, and heavy metals.

Famotidine: A peptic agent that treats stomach acid, ulcers, gastro-esophageal reflux, and assists with nausea control.

Ketorolac: The generic of brand name Toradol, Ketorolac is a non-steroidal anti-inflammatory drug used to treat aches, pains, and headaches.

Ondansetron: The generic form of brand name Zofran, Ondansetron is an anti-nausea med, which unlike other popular anti-nausea meds does not cause drowsiness. You'll get 30, or sometimes 60, milligrams, which taken intravenously is PLENTY.

Triamino: Often referred to as OAC, Triamino is a blend of three strong amino acids (Ornithine, Arginine, and Citroline) which increase metabolic rate and assist in muscular repair after athletic activity.

Zinc: A trace mineral that is known to shorten the length of the common cold and other viral infections, zinc is included in a lot of "cold remedy" IVs.

Vitamin D: Great for the immune system, and critical for the absorption of calcium. Vitamin D is an injection given separate from IV therapy.

NAD+ (Nicotinamide Adenine Dinucleotide):

Put simply, Nicotinamide Adenine Dinucleotide (NAD+) is a "cofactor" in cellular metabolism. A "cofactor" is a molecule (chemical compound) necessary for an enzyme to function. It's called a "dinucleotide" because it's a group of two nucleotides (one is nicotinamide and the other is an adenine nucleobase) which are joined together by a phosphate group. You can think of it as a double railcar joined together with a link, that moves material from one station to another to allow the work at the receiving station to progress.

The simplest way to put what NAD+ is/does is that it moves electrons from Point A to Point B, so the station at Point B can use the electrons to perform a job. NAD+ "picks up" a Hydrogen molecule (one electron), becomes NADH, then essentially deposits the electron and becomes NAD+ again. The electron is now in the mitochondria (remember your teacher calling it the "power plant of the cell"?), helps generate ATP, and the product created is used to power the specific function of the cell.

NAD is becoming very popular with IV centers around the country, but if you're going to get it make SURE they do a thorough screening on you, and that you're prepared for the possibility of immediate, noticeable physiological effects (chest tightening, warm sensation, etc.).

A "Banana Bag": What's a banana bag? Well, there's a question everyone thinks has a simple answer, which really doesn't.

Believe it or not, there's no "rule" or "regulation" about what can be called a banana bag, or what something called a banana bag has to include. MOST reputable medical facilities don't call anything a banana bag with regularity (at least officially), unless they have a stated procedure about it. However, almost all places that infuse something they call a banana bag include at least three things: folic acid (vitamin B9), thiamine (vitamin B1), and magnesium, and most include a low-potency multivitamin.

In general, in a hospital setting banana bags are given to chronic alcoholics, people who have had weight loss surgery, terminally ill patients, or those who have experienced a temporary physical issue that has led to loss of fluids and caused physical pain.

Thiamine is included in banana bags, among other reasons, to prevent a syndrome called Wernicke's Disease, which affects both long term alcohol abusers and those who have had weight loss surgery. It's also used to fight the effects of a deficiency caused by a diet that doesn't include enough grains and/or legumes. Both issues are prevalent in those two demographics, and can lead to Wernicke's (which can cause vision issues up to and including blindness). It's VERY effective for people who haven't eaten properly, who (like many of us in the South) eat a mostly meat-centered diet, or who have skipped meals regularly.

Folic acid (the manufactured form of Folate, or B9) is used to fight anemia. It's also required by the body for RNA and DNA production and cellular division. It can't be made BY the body, so it HAS to be absorbed through food. Those who haven't gotten proper nutrition are subject to Folic acid deficiency, which can lead to abnormally enlarged red blood cells, and a host of issues. Chronic tiredness, heart palpitations (atrial fibrillation and atrial flutter), and an increased risk of stroke are all possibilities when someone is folic deficient.

Magnesium is a natural muscle relaxant that works wonders with muscle cramps, spasms, tremors, muscle pain, and heart palpitations.

Because most people who need a banana bag haven't, at least recently, been managing a well-balanced diet, a low-potency multivitamin that includes a few B vitamins is also usually included.

Last, but not least, everyone asks why the banana bag is called that, and what makes it yellow. Many people mistakenly assume that potassium in the bag turns the fluids yellow, because they know bananas are high in potassium and think that potassium must be what makes them both yellow. As you now know, most banana bags have no potassium at all. It's the multivitamin that makes the bag yellow. The name comes from the yellow color, not from any particular ingredient.

Now you know what a banana bag is. Anyone can call any IV bag full of fluids that turns yellow a "banana bag". Before you get one anywhere make sure you ask EXACTLY what's in your bag.

"Myers Cocktail": You've heard the term "Myers' Cocktail" for the better part of your adult life. It's said to be anything from a complete waste of time and money to a magic mixture of medicines in an IV bag that can cure whatever ails you.

So, before we can talk about the pros and cons of the treatment, it's important to know what's in it. What's the "recipe" for a Myers' Cocktail and what are the "ingredients" in it intended to do?

Well, it may shock you to know that nobody knows exactly. That's right. John Myers, M.D., the doctor who initially "created" the concoction that became known as the Myers' Cocktail never bothered to write down his recipe. As a matter of fact, while giving the treatment at Johns Hopkins (world-famous hospital in Baltimore, Maryland where my Grandpa was actually Chief of Cardio-Thoracic Surgery) Myers never even named it. His colleague Dr. Alan Gaby attempted to recreate the formulae after Myers passed away, and named it "Myers' Cocktail" as a tribute. Even the guy who named it doesn't know what Myers put in it. It's assumed he often changed the additives and concentrations based on what was available, and what a specific patient may need. There's no set rule about what can be called a Myers' Cocktail, what you have to put in it, or what you can add to the common mixture.

Seems crazy doesn't it? If you order a "bourbon and Coke" you know you're getting bourbon, and Coke. If you ask for a Myers' Cocktail the only way you're going to know what's in it is if you ask for the specifics, and two places sharing the same parking lot may have two wildly different "recipes".

In MOST Myers' Cocktails you see marketed by IV centers in The United States, you'll find a few main ingredients:

* **B-complex vitamins**
* **Vitamin C**
* **Magnesium Chloride (or magnesium sulfate)**
* **Calcium gluconate**

So, why IV, and why those ingredients? For starters, you probably know by now that anything you take IV is immediately "bioavailable", meaning your body starts using it/reacting to it immediately. Anything that you consume orally is going to take time to get through your system to the point that your actual cells and organs can make use of it. Worse, the majority of what you consume orally is not absorbed, it's passed and is never put to use.

How about those ingredients? Why them?

*B-complex vitamins: These are a bit of a "trick" in my opinion. Very few people in the developed world suffer from B vitamin deficiencies. Usually this is restricted to those on extreme diets, or people who have had gastric sleeve or bypass surgery. Though B-complex can do wonders for people with chronic anemia and other "failure to thrive" issues, for the bulk of us, it's simply a "pick me up". You'll get a boost similar to several cups of coffee, or one of those nasty energy drinks. You aren't deficient in any of the B vitamins in all likelihood, but you will feel a little extra pep in your step. It's strictly conjecture on my part, but I feel like putting this in when it's not necessary had to be part of a plan to have people say "I did Dr. Myers' magic IV and I felt like a million bucks when it was over". Of course you did, because you got a stimulant. IF that's what you're looking for, great, but don't be fooled that all the little vitamins and minerals have suddenly made you "extra healthy". You're feeling great because you just got injected with Go Juice.

*Vitamin C: This is the ingredient that is the reason so many people with various forms of arthritis or fibromyalgia swear by the Myers' Cocktail. Vitamin C is a fantastic anti-inflammatory. Much of what causes pain in joints and soft tissues can be traced back to inflammation. So, while they're getting a little energy from the B-complex, the Vitamin C is working to reduce the inflammation in their joints and soft tissues. Some IV places will put a dose of Toradol (or the generic form called Ketorolac), which is a non-steroidal anti-inflammatory like Advil, in with the Vitamin C to give temporary pain relief to give the more intermediate term anti-inflammatory Vitamin C time to work. That's sort of cheating, but if it works to relieve the pain of the patient, more power to them.

*Magnesium: Usually this is Magnesium Chloride, though it's sometimes Magnesium Sulfate, which is generally less expensive and more readily available. Mag Chloride is really only distributed by one producer in the U.S. and it can get tricky to acquire. That aside, the magnesium (in any form) is included because it's a fairly strong natural muscle relaxant. It certainly helps with pain, and just as importantly lets the Vitamin C work its way into the areas it need to be to reduce inflammation.

*Calcium gluconate: Oddly, calcium gluconate is a compound that is used to treat magnesium poisoning in the blood, so there's some thought that maybe this was included as a precaution. The better guess is that because many of the people who have poor enough dietary habits to need additional magnesium, B vitamins, and vitamin C, also lack calcium in their diet, this was included to reverse the effects of hypocalcemia. Many conditions like Rickets and osteoarthritis are amplified when osteoporosis sets in as a consequence of low calcium intake.

So there is your list of the common ingredients in a Myers' Cocktail. Increasingly today you'll see other things added as well. Glutathione is becoming widely used, even though the powerful antioxidant hadn't even been isolated and produced before Myers' death. Glutathione is great for liver health, cellular restoration, and several other things, but it wasn't part of the original concoction for those suffering from various inflammatory/degenerative conditions. Putting peaches and raisins in Grandma's apple pie recipe might taste great, but then it isn't really Grandma's apple pie is it?

Zinc: known to shorten the duration of respiratory illnesses, has also become a frequent addition to the Myers'.

The point of all this "what's in it" discussion is that if you care about what you're getting, you REALLY need to look at the list of ingredients in a facility's Myers' Cocktail before you get infused with it. They aren't all the same.

So, what is a Myers' Cocktail really good for, and when is it a waste of time?

First shot out of the box, let's talk about the elephant in the room. Cancer. If anyone tells you that a Myers' Cocktail regimen can cure cancer, they're either telling you what they think is true and they're simply completely deluded, or they're lying to you. I read once a week that there's some IV that can cure cancer. Pardon my language, but that's bullshit. To be completely honest, we love helping people, but we aren't running a charity. If there were an IV that cured cancer we'd be lining people up at the door, selling it by the pallet, and buying vacation homes. Some places do put glutathione in their Myers', and there have been studies (though I can't speak to their methods or scientific rigor) that have shown some success keeping tumors from growing with glutathione, but that doesn't mean that getting a tiny amount of it every other week in a Myers' Cocktail is going to cure cancer.

I'm a big fan of the Myers for people with arthritis, whether it's rheumatoid arthritis, osteoarthritis, or otherwise. The calcium obviously helps with bone health. The Vitamin C is great for slowing the inflammation that comes with arthritis (remember, "itis" means, in essence, swelling). The magnesium is a muscle relaxant that enhances the efficacy of the C, and provides a natural pain-relieving factor by relieving muscle tension. The B-complex gives a nice boost.

Similarly, all the anti-inflammatory and muscle relaxing properties of a Myers' make it a winner for people with asthma. Lessening inflammation in the lungs, and relaxing the airway are winners for those folks. If you have asthma you know what we're talking about.

A Myers is also great for fibromyalgia, chronic fatigue, colds, and other similar conditions. It's not going to keep you from aging, and it's not going to cure your cancer. It's a great treatment for those who have very specific issues but you can't walk into an IV center as a 67 year old with cancer, get a Myers' Cocktail, and walk out like a 52 year old who's in remission.

Dextrose: Typically this comes in 1 liter bags of fluid as "5%", which equates to 50mL of 50% dextrose in a 1L bag. Many people get dextrose when they're hypoglycemic (low blood sugar), but it should be avoided for most diabetics as it can cause a spike in blood sugar. Only a few IV centers will give dextrose, as the complications can be intense.

Vitamin B12:   There are some crazy claims about B12 on the internet. Most are unfounded. While it is true that B12 is essential in cellular metabolism, red blood cell production, nerve function, and the production of DNA.

We think of it as a natural version of one of those energy shots. Though you can end up with a form of anemia from a B12 deficiency, it's really incredibly rare. The half-life of B12 is quite literally years in your body. There's not much of a chance that you're B12 deficient, though it does give you a nice boost either way.

Claims that B12 prevent heart disease are based on old studies, long since disproven. Take it for what it is; a nice little boost when taken responsibly and occasionally.

Biotin: B7 (biotin) is in just about every "beauty" IV you see advertised, anywhere. All the claims of nail and hair strengthening, and skin improvement are based on a single, pre-clinical study, conducted several decades ago without placebo controls, that concluded participants' nails were "less brittle" after a multi-week oral regimen of B7, and a study that showed at least a perception of a "healthy glow" in skin. Biotin is known to be essential in the health of cow's hooves, which leads everyone back to the hair, skin, and nail claims. Though likely unnecessary, it's very easily absorbed and processed so there's little to no chance of harm from receiving biotin, but it's not the Fountain of Youth.

CHAPTER 5:

What are Some of the Risks of Getting IV Therapy?

That's a question we get asked quite a bit, and people seem to expect us to say "nothing really". Wouldn't that be great? "No risk at all." We'd love to be able to say that, but it's simply not true. Granted, you may be at just as much risk driving to the office, but nothing is without risk, especially not something involving an (and I was told not to use this word) invasive medical procedure (I was told not to use that word either, but honesty is the best policy).

So, let's look at the possible negative effects of getting an IV, and let's talk about how to avoid them.

1) Infection: Let's just start off with the biggie. Nationally, you probably see this quite a bit. It doesn't happen at our IV center (Rapid Recovery) for very specific reasons, but it does happen elsewhere. Someone is about to insert a needle into your vein. Whatever is on that needle is going into your bloodstream. Make sure they are wearing gloves, they don't sneeze, they clean the infusion site VERY well before inserting the catheter, and you are in a clean environment. That's a good start.

More important is what happens AFTER your infusion is over. At Rapid Recovery we give you an AfterCare card, and it's not a joke or something cool to show your friends. It has an alcohol swab and a bandaid attached to it. You're going to leave with a clean infusion site and some form of bandage over the area where you got your IV. Fantastic. That's gonna work really well for a few hours, or until you start sweating a lot. The reason we give you the bandaid and the alcohol swab is that eventually you're going to need to change that bandage. Remove it in a clean area, clean the site well with the alcohol swab we gave you, and replace the bandage with the new one.

If your chosen IV center doesn't offer a change of bandage and an alcohol swab, be sure to grab one yourself. A nasty bandage that has gotten sweat and/or dirt on the underside where your infusion site is can be a real infection risk. Make sure you change that bandage.

If you're at a clean IV center and you use some common sense after leaving, you shouldn't get an infection.

In the rare case that you start noticing swelling, heat around your infusion area, and redness, you may be getting the beginning of an infection. Wherever you got your IV, contact them immediately.

2) Allergic reaction: If you've ever been to our place, when you got your first IV we made you fill out a LONG allergy questionnaire. That wasn't just to waste your time. When you have an allergy, be it to niacin, large doses of folic acid, maybe magnesium sensitivity, and you get that thing infused directly into your blood stream, you're going to have an issue. That's why you need to only go to IV centers that are very serious about your allergy history. You'll also notice that at better IV centers your IV specialist hovers over you like an annoying waiter for the first several minutes of your infusion. If you're going to have an allergic reaction to something, when that something is pumping right into your bloodstream it's going to happen pretty quickly. So you want to go to a place that will wait to make sure nothing is going to happen.

Please, for the love of God and baseball, don't gloss over your allergy questionnaire or lie on it because you think it's "not a big deal". Sometimes, in really rare instances when someone gets something they don't KNOW they're allergic to, you'll experience anaphylaxis from something or other. Don't panic. Most IV centers keep Benadryl and Epinephrine on hand for those rare cases.

In most cases they'll discontinue the "loaded" IV, replace it with a plain solution of Ringer's Lactate (or sodium chloride), and hit you with a quick fix of Benadryl.

3) Kidney stones: This one is counterintuitive isn't it? It seems like you get fluids and stay hydrated to KEEP FROM GETTING kidney stones. Well, turns out that if you get really large doses of Vitamin C, such that your kidneys can't process it, you might end up with a kidney stone. That's part of the reason that we don't give more than 10 grams of Vitamin C.

People who don't process calcium well may also be at risk for developing a kidney stone. The trick is that getting any of these vitamins or minerals in a liter of fluids generally takes that risk down to almost nothing, UNLESS you have kidney issues. Most professional IV centers have a pretty strict policy regarding treating anyone who has any kidney issues, and if you've had any lack of kidney function they won't infuse you with anything other than fluids without specific instructions from your Nephrologist.

If you even HAVE a nephrologist, be sure to let your IV center know it, and let them know about any kidney issues you've had.

4) Birth defects: As a former neonatal specialist, I'm absolutely paranoid about birth defects. Though some centers will (as we've discussed) we simply don't treat anyone who is pregnant without very specific instructions from their current, treating Obstetrician. Blood pressure issues, fetal heart rate being affected, etc., can be serious and many centers prefer to simply stay away from any possible complications, for your safety and the safety of your baby. Some will, if EVERYTHING is just right and your OB says it's okay, give you fluids, but it's unlikely that any will give Zofran (Ondansetron) or other additives to pregnant women.

5) Phlebitis: This is one you should Google. Pretty rare, but it does cause redness, swelling, and pain. It happens when an IV is inserted improperly. How rare is this? Not as rare as you'd hope. It doesn't happen at our place because we only hire RNs with at least 5 years of intensive IV experience. By intensive we mean ER, ICU, or other places where a huge chunk of what they do is start IVs. But, it does happen at some IV centers. Why? Inexperience.

6) Cardiovascular distress: If you are at an IV place, even if you've been a dozen times, and they don't take your pulse and your blood pressure, get the hell out of there as quickly as you politely can.

Some meds, and even just fluids in general, can cause fluctuations in your pulse and BP. Imagine you're sitting at 80 over 60 (which is really low), and something in your bag, say magnesium, can cause a rapid drop in blood pressure. Now imagine that your nurse doesn't bother to take your BP before starting your infusion. That doesn't sound great does it?

What if your resting pulse is normally 72-80, but for some reason you're at 112 and your nurse/IV specialist doesn't know it because they didn't take a pulse. Then they start an infusion that has a stimulant of some nature in it, and your pulse spikes.

Cardiovascular problems are possible, but the chances of having them are significantly reduced if you're within normal parameters and someone checks to make sure. And remember, "I feel fine" doesn't cut it.

There are other risks associated with IV therapy, and we could talk about them all day, but the best way to reduce the risk is to (1) go to a reputable IV therapy center, (2) make sure they take your medical history the first time you go, (3) make sure they check your vitals EVERY time you get an IV, (4) follow their instructions for infusion site care, and (5) always be honest with your provider about allergies and other known conditions. Basically, the real answer to "is it safe" is "yes, if you do what you're supposed to do, and go to a place where they do what they're supposed to do as well."

CHAPTER 6:

Where Should I Get IV Therapy?

If you're looking for a name and an address, that's coming later. For now, let's talk about things to seek out in an IV center, things to be scared of, and questions to ask.

Remember, just because something is common and generally safe doesn't mean you should do it just anywhere. Think about something like bungee jumping, or better yet, zip-lining. There are hundreds of safe, reputable places where you can go on a zipline adventure. You know Place A. Ads all over town. They have new or like-new harnesses, they train their employees well, the owner is around to make sure things go the way they should, the person strapping you in has the most experience of anyone on the team and there's a younger kid learning from them, the lines are checked regularly and are 5 times as strong as they need to be, etc., etc., etc.

Then you've got Place B. The harness looks a little worn, but it's probably still safe. The metal zipline has a little rust on it, but that's likely not an issue. They've been pretty busy so the kid who straps you into the harness isn't quite a pro, but that's why there are safety straps, right?

Forget it. There's still a chance something will go wrong at Place A, but not nearly as great a chance that something will at Place B. You see, Place A is professional. Place B is a business, but that doesn't make it professional.

So with that in mind, let's look at some of the things you need to look for in an IV therapy center, some of the things you'll want to steer clear of, and some of the things you should run like hell from.

1)   The website.

No, I'm not saying you need to go to a place that has a fancy website because I think having a fancy website means it's a great company.

I'm talking about information, transparency, and hyperbole.

Information:

For starters, is there REAL information about what you're getting?

There's no special widget that one IV center can get that another can't. This isn't like Coke and Pepsi. They're all serving Coke in some form or fashion, or they all CAN serve Coke. No such thing as an exclusive. Anything IV World can get, Hydration Station can get. So the whole "protecting our secret formula" doesn't exist. The question is, are they telling you exactly what's in the fluids you're having infused?

You don't want to land at a place that has a beautiful website with names of packages like "the Jetlag Buster", but doesn't tell you what's in the bag of fluids. If they don't say, they may not even KNOW. A lot of these places buy their "packages" from national pharmacies or IV fulfillment centers, and simply slap a logo sticker on the bag and give it a trendy name.

What you want to look for is a place that has a nice little write-up on their hangover package or their food poisoning package, or whatever package, that tells you exactly what's in that bag of fluids, and why you need it. If nothing else, this tells you that they're familiar with their own offerings and aren't getting them from a wholesale operation.

On the topic of information, you'd like to see some original content.

Do these people know their own business well enough to write about it intelligently, or are they just poking people with needles because it's supposed to be a profitable business? If they have a section of their website devoted to their own videos where they describe their IVs, or an original blog section where they go into all the details of their Myers' Cocktail or their Immune Defender (or whatever they call it), you know that THEY KNOW what they're talking about. Look for a weekly or monthly health tip or explanation video or post that they wrote themselves (you can tell), and if you find it you'll know you've got someone who is dedicated to not only learning about their own craft, but teaching you as well.

Transparency:

This is a big one that often goes overlooked. Transparency on a website is, once again, indicative of professionalism.

Do they tell you the prices? If not, why not? Do they just want you to come in and then feel committed to getting an IV even if it's higher than you think it should be? Are they charging more at one location than another? Do they want you to call so they can talk you into it?

You wouldn't show up at Best Buy for a TV if the website didn't have the price on it.

Here's another transparency issue: Who's in charge? Is there an "About Us" page that tells you who the owners are, what their level of involvement is, what their protocols are, who their doctor is, and similar information?

Think about it. Jane works in home health and her husband is an insurance salesman. He makes a good amount of money and they have some savings. She's tired of her job and knows a Nurse Practitioner (Mary) who will take $500 a month to sign their prescriptions. Mary is supervised by an Orthopedic Surgeon who hasn't given an IV ever, and doesn't know much (if anything) about what goes in one, even though he or she is a great surgeon.

So Jane whips up an IV spa. She buys packages from a pharmacy in Florida, and Mary signs the orders. What the hell kind of system is that? Not a safe one.

Make sure there's transparency on their website and that you know who is in charge and how they're running things.

Hyperbole:

"Burn belly fat while you sleep", "Look 10 years younger", "Proven to Shrink Tumors", "Reverse the Effects of Aging"… if you see anything like that on an IV center's website, and you REALLY want to try the place, you better go now before the Food and Drug Administration shuts them down for false claims. It has happened, and it will happen again.

What you want to see on an IV spa's website is some sort of credible information explaining what each med/vitamin/ingredient/additive is intended to do for you, and some research in an FAQ section or information section that backs up those claims. For example, "our Arthritis Package is loaded with Vitamin C, glucosamine, and chondroitin," is okay if they have an explanation about the anti-inflammatory effects of C, and the joint lubrication functions of glucosamine and chondroitin.

Nothing takes ten years off your face, nothing at an IV spa cures cancer, and nothing burns belly fat while you sleep. Look for a website that is clear, concise, honest in its claims, and provides real information. We're talking about a medical procedure here, not a magic elixir.

2) The Office

First off, do they have their own dedicated office? If they don't, they might be winging it. You want to walk into a clean, well-appointed office that's in a decent part of town, which looks like a place you'd be happy to own.

If the place you're considering is well-lit, has employees in company logo apparel, a nice sign, clean floors, a legit brochure/menu, and quality furnishings there's a good chance they care about the way you're treated.

That's not to say that you can judge a book by its cover, it's just saying that a well-kept, quality environment is generally indicative of an organization that cares. If they take good care of their office, there's a much better chance they're going to take good care of you.

3) The Walls

What? The walls? Yeah, sort of. Look on the walls. Do you see a Medical License posted for the physician? Do you see a Health Department (if required by their state) license posted? Do you see tax license posted if they sell merchandise?

Some of these items aren't required in some places, but a Physician License should be conspicuously displayed in the office, and if it isn't that generally means the IV center doesn't know the regulations, which is scary, or the physician doesn't want their license plastered up on the wall, and that's equally scary.

Look for a HIPAA (Health Insurance Portability and Accountability Act) notice, and make sure you signed one. Any legitimate medical facility will have posted their HIPAA Compliance Notice, make it available for you to read, ask you to sign one, and give you a copy if you want one.

4)   The Prep Room or Med Room

Some of the better IV centers, and I'm thinking of Health Hydration Oasis in Milwaukee right now, have windows that look into their IV preparation room. Super cool that you can actually watch them mix your bag without even being in the room. Corey Garrett Brown at Elevation Hydration mixes bags right in front of you.

At the very least, ask if you are allowed to see the area where they create your IV. Is it tidy? Do they work on a stainless steel (easily disinfected) surface? Is the nurse gloved while preparing your bag? Do you see a red (biohazard) trashcan? Is there a thermometer attached to the medicine fridge, with a temperature log next to it?

If an IV spa is doing things the right way they shouldn't be at all concerned about you watching them prepare your IV. After all, it's going into your bloodstream, right?

If you look into a prep area and it's disorganized, dirty, or doesn't feel "clean and safe", then you probably don't want them preparing a solution that's about to go straight into your system.

5)   The staff

Nothing against young people, I wish I were young again so I wouldn't ache everywhere, all the time, but you want experience in your IV staff.

My Dad is an Obstetrician and he's kind of the guru of obstetrics. Even when he's not on call, other doctors, sometimes not even obstetricians, will ask him for advice on tricky patients, or ask him to come to the hospital to assist or take over a scary surgery. I asked him once how the hell he knows so much. He said simply "I've been doing it for a LONG time. You might only see something once a decade, so somebody who's been at it for 8 or 9 year might never have seen it. I've seen it 4 or 5 times so it's old hat."

An experienced ICU, ER, or OB nurse, or longtime EMT/ paramedic, has started quite literally thousands of IVs. Most of them in really tough to stick patients, and sometimes under incredibly trying circumstances. Imagine, someone is rushed into an ER after a gunshot, they have no anesthesia on board, they're flopping around in pain, and you're asked to start an IV, and by God it needs to be in them NOW. Well after a few years of that, or trying to hit a vein in an ambulance on a bumpy road, getting an IV in someone who's sitting in a lounge chair in a quiet IV spa seems like child's play.

I always think of it like warfare. Give me the person who has been in battle, a lot, when the bullets start flying.

Some places hire the youngest, cutest or buffest, perkiest employees for the look of it. Great. Give me that old person who hobbles into my room and knows exactly what they're doing.

Here's another something: What if, Lord forbid, something goes wrong? You have an allergic reaction, or you blow a vein or something. Well that experienced IV specialist has seen it plenty of times, and there's no panic in them. The younger employee might have a fit. We've had a few bad situations. We had a drug abuser lie on a form and start losing their mind as soon as the fluids started going into their system. It had nothing to do with the IV. They were getting fluids and vitamins. Luckily our nurse was incredibly experienced, knew exactly what the score was, didn't panic, and handled the situation like a pro.

We've had it with allergic reactions as well. The more experienced nurses know to discontinue the IV, start a bag of straight fluids, administer some Benadryl, and help the patient calm down.

Experience. It counts.

6)   Materials

The materials matter. Really. Are they using Becton Dickinson IV catheters, or just whatever they can get on the internet for a bargain basement price?

Are their drugs all from reputable U.S. based pharmacies or wholesale vendors, or are they buying whatever they can for ½ price that says "Myers' Cocktail" on it? Do they have a sharps container in every room?

An IV center is no different than any other worksite. If they don't have the right tools, they can't do the job the way it's meant to be done.

7)   Technology

Believe it or not, this is HUGE. You wouldn't think it, but it is.

Now you're curious.

So, let's say you show up at an IV center and the intake person hands you a clipboard to fill out your initial visit paperwork. You mark down that you're a person who gets niacin flush. It's a fairly uncommon, but not unseen, condition that sends your pulse and blood pressure straight to the moon, causes chest pain, and really freaks you out. It's really easily reversed so there's no reason to be worried, but it could be avoided.

How did it happen? The IV starter didn't dig through all your paperwork because it was six sheets of paper. If they had an electronic system, when they went to enter what you're getting the system would've said "nope". A good center has a software package (even if, like IVme in Chicago, they built it themselves) that would stop someone from giving you something your medical questionnaire showed was contraindicated.

Worse, what happens the second time you come in and have a different nurse/IV starter? Is that person going to go through your chart to make sure you're not supposed to have X, Y, or Z? Probably not, and guess what's going to happen. Just one guess.

Here's another scary scenario. You get an IV on Saturday, and it's got a bunch of ketorolac in it. You're feeling a little beat Sunday after playing tennis all day, so you come in for another. The nurse asks if you've ever been in before, you say yes, and off they go. Uh-oh. Really bad for your liver to be getting ketorolac again, but it's a different IV starter, you don't know that, and their system doesn't say "wait a minute".

Paper is something that everyone does for about a month when they're starting out and they haven't mastered the system. If you see paper, either the IV center is brand new (and that's scary), or they just plain don't have the best available technology (and that's scary as well).

8) After the IV

When you're done, and your IV center employee removes your IV and puts a bandage on you, do they wave and say goodbye, or do they do something else?

At a credible IV center, you'll get a bandage change. Your bandage isn't going to last that long, especially if you live in the South and get your IV in the summer. Whatever they put on you is going to get dirty and/or sweaty and you might not have what you need to replace it lying around. To keep from getting an infection you're going to need to replace it. Hopefully you're at a center that cares.

Did they give you anything that details what they infused into you? What if your doctor asks tomorrow? Are you going to tell them to look up the website? What if you aren't feeling great in a week and want to review what you got last time? Most of the more well-organized IV centers will give you something on paper, or send you an email, that details everything they gave you.

9) Reviews... sometimes...

Take a close look at the reviews of a place before you decide to let them infuse you. If they have more than one location, it's okay to look at the other locations as well.

There might be a bad review here and there. That's okay. There's always some crazy person who walks into a place expecting the moon and loses it when they don't get it. Look at the preponderance of the sentiment from their patients. Look and see if they have any regulars.

Check Google and Facebook. Look at the comments on their posts, the number of people who've checked-in, everything.

While you're at it, look to see that the reviews are organic. There are lots of new services that will drag reviews out of people, and curate them so you only see the good ones. Worthless.

10.   Bigger isn't always better

I'm not talking about the office building. I'm talking about the organization.

Now, that isn't to say that a huge company can't be great. I remember seeing a Budweiser ad (in case you don't know, Budweiser sells more "Bud" – the regular one – every year than has ever been sold all-time of most any other beer you can name) and it said "we used to be a microbrew too". The implication there was that once a ton of people had tasted Bud, they all started buying it. So, they had to make more because it's that damned good...

So, back to IV centers... If a company has an ad (or website) that says they have 48 locations in 13 states, are they concerned about staying on top of quality, about making sure every employee is giving 100% all the time, or are they focusing on "corporate profits"?

You can't talk in absolutes, and the biggest may be the best, but in general if I'm talking about my health I want a local person whose reputation depends on doing things the right way, who I'm going to see at a restaurant, whose kids go to school with my daughter, who I KNOW is as interested in my health as they are in their profits.

CHAPTER 7:

What to Avoid When Looking for an IV Center

Just as important as knowing what to look for in an IV center is knowing what to avoid like the plague.

We've discussed a lot of these things in previous topics, but they bear repeating if so, and certainly need to be covered if we haven't so far.

1) Custom or common?

If you don't have any allergies, aren't particularly sensitive to anything, don't react oddly to anything, and don't mind paying for something you don't need, maybe this isn't as big a deal for you as it is for others. If any of those apply to you, maybe it matters.

The better IV centers mix their IV treatments "from scratch". Chains and questionable places buy either the bags already premixed (and refrigerate them), or buy the "IV in a bottle" and just inject it into their base fluid.

Again, maybe fine as long as their migraine package doesn't have magnesium, and you're sensitive to it. Maybe fine as long as you don't get niacin flush and their hangover bag is loaded with it.

It's an oversimplification, but what if all Super Burgers came with mustard, and you just don't like mustard on your burger? Would you go to Super Burger anyway and suffer through the mustard or would you go somewhere they'd give you what you want? Burger King dug into McDonald's business in a big way with their "Have it Your Way" ad campaign. They knew a long time ago, custom is better than pre-packaged.

Stay away from chains that mail their treatments to local places, and anyone who buys their treatments in a bottle from a pharmacy that supplies everyone with the same pre-mixed "treatment in a bottle". These are more common than you'd think. If you go to their website and it says "yourtown. megacorp.com", there's a good chance they're sending six of these and nine of these and 5 of those to their satellite office and telling them what to recommend. "We're running a special on those Pump It Up IVs because we mailed out 100 last week and they're about to expire, so run a Facebook ad for 15 bucks off to get rid of them."

Don't even ask if they mix every bag themselves. Ask if you can leave _____ out of their _____ IV. You'll know what you're dealing with if you do.

2)   Attitude

This is going to sound ridiculous, but hear me out. What's the place named? It matters.

Why does it matter? A name reflects the attitude, and their level of seriousness about the operation.

A place called Hangover Busters, IV Bar, Dr. Buzz, or anything similar, isn't likely treating this like a medical procedure, they're treating it like a joke or a casual deal. You might be in a lounge setting with a big leather recliner, or a pink chaise, or even in a beanbag, but you're getting a needle stuck in you and something piped into your bloodstream. Do you really want the people at Hangover Helper performing a medical procedure on you?

3)   Though not always, mobile-only IV services

It costs about four hundred bucks to incorporate an LLC. It costs a little more to make sure you protect your personal assets in the event something goes wrong. That's not much of an "all-in" investment. If something goes horribly wrong, the company gets bankrupted and the owner forms another.

An office, with a lease or a mortgage, a bunch of furniture, an expensive sign, all with the owner's name and personal guarantee on them, indicate a level of commitment.

The person who remodeled an old warehouse with their life's savings, signed a 5 year lease on a place downtown (with a personal guarantee), and who maxed out their Visa card on oxygen concentrators and IV supplies, they're in it for good and they're going to do it the right way.

That isn't to say there aren't GREAT mobile-only IV companies. There's a company based out of El Paso, Texas (Drip Drive) that does mobile-only in Waco, Texas, and they're fabulous. There's an outstanding mobile-only service (Drip Dynamics) in Houston. If you don't know for sure though, tie goes to the runner. Take the place, and the owner, that's all-in.

4)   Questionable medical director/direction

It's completely appropriate to ask (or look at the website of) an IV center about their medical director.

Some of the better centers around the country, like Hydrate Medical in Charlotte, North Carolina, and the previously mentioned Health Hydration Oasis, actually have their doctors on site.

This is very important: A good IV center will have an Internal Medicine physician, an Anesthesiologist, an Infectious Disease specialist, an Endocrinologist, or an ER doc, as their Medical Director.

Why? These are people who have experience with IVs and/or understand a broad array of medical conditions. They're "doctors", not highly specialized people who are epic at one thing (like brain surgery), but unfamiliar with daily health issues.

Nothing against chiropractors, but they can't even prescribe medicines in most states (if not all), and they actually usually have a medical doctor reviewing some of their work. I just can't see getting a prescription item from someone who reports to a nurse practitioner, who reports to a chiropractor, who reports to a family practitioner, who has no idea what the hell is going on at that IV center.

If you find out that the place you're considering has an orthopedic surgeon as a medical director, let me tell you a quick story.

I work with Orthos. Love most of them. Once an Ortho I know was in an exam room going over an upcoming surgery with a patient, and the patient had a heart attack. The Ortho comes running out of the room and screams, "We need a doctor here!" His staff looked at him confused and said "Eddie, you ARE a doctor." His response was "I mean a REAL doctor."

You see where I'm going with that? Psychiatrists, Orthopedists, Chiropractors, Obstetricians, Urologists... I could go on.

There are thousands upon thousands of them who might be smarter than 99% of the medical directors of IV centers, but they're specialized in something that doesn't matter in the field you're asking to serve you. I wouldn't get my broken bones or torn ligaments treated by an Endocrinologist, and I wouldn't get my IV therapy at a place whose medical director is an Ortho.

I humbly assert that I'm damned good at my job, and I probably do a lot of things pretty well, but if you dropped me in a Taco Bell tomorrow morning I would absolutely mangle every burrito I tried to make. Just because I can turn around a physician's practice or run a business doesn't mean I know a damned thing about making an enchilada. Same principle.

Stay away from questionable or unrelated medical direction.

5)   Bad infection prevention procedures

First off, if you walk into an IV center and they put you in a room that's dirty, stand back up and leave.

If you see a wrapper from a safety needle on the ground, IV tubing in a regular trashcan (because there's likely blood in it), or a used nasal cannula (from an oxygen concentrator), you're in the wrong place.

If your nurse shows up to start your IV and isn't wearing gloves, game over.

If at all possible, before booking your appointment look up your potential center online (Facebook, YouTube, their website, etc.) and see if there are any write-ups or videos of their infection control procedures. If there are, you're probably in good shape.

You'll likely have a gut feeling. The place is either serious about infection control, or it isn't, and it will probably be obvious. Don't stay anywhere you aren't comfortable.

6)   More than a few bad reviews

Like I said earlier, there are always crazy people. You've dealt with them in your job. Some irrational person who complains when there really isn't reason to complain. If you see one of those, or even a few, it's probably not a big deal, especially if you see a bunch of great reviews.

If, though, you see more than one review like "they tried to hit my vein 4 times and couldn't", or "my appointment started 30 minutes late and they didn't apologize or offer a discount", or "they couldn't really explain what was in the different packages", then maybe you're at the wrong place.

Out of thousands of patients, every IV center is going to have a few loud whackos who want to cause trouble on the internet. Not every center is going to have several, and the ones which do are probably not worth visiting.

7)   Jack of All Trades

Have you ever seen those places that have signs that say "Auto Insurance, Tax Filing, Notary, Money Orders"?

Would you really let someone who sells money orders and car insurance prepare your taxes? Probably not. Likewise, I wouldn't buy my car insurance from a notary.

We see the most unbelievable places offering to give you an IV. My personal favorite is hair salons. They're probably doing one or two IVs a day. That's the place to go if you need a color or a trim, but it simply can't be a good idea to get a medical procedure done at a place that's more worried about highlights than hydration.

Several "med spas" around the country are heading in this direction. They'll do stem cell injections, hormone replacement, sono/laser/electro "fat blasting", cryotherapy, IVs, Botox, Juviderm, facials, massages, and everything under the sun. They're usually beautiful facilities, and they have all the trappings of greatness. The problem is that they just aren't experts at any of it. We (Rapid Recovery) have two nurses who are certified to give Botox injections, and we could make a killing doing it, but we'll NEVER be as good as Fixx Med Spa because it's what they do. They could add IVs, but they'll never be able to follow all the procedures we do, or be as safe, or as good, as we are because they're all we do. So we both stay in our lane.

There are a few notable exceptions, but they're rare. There's usually one nurse who does Botox in a good IV spa that offers it, and it's usually not even done every day.

I've got a buddy named Larry West who owns an outstanding cryospa (Chill & Heal) in Shreveport, Louisiana. A Cryospa is one of those places they put you in a tube and fire liquid nitrogen (or something) into the tube and lower the temperature around your body to something like minus 200 degree Fahrenheit for like 60 seconds. In the same building with him was an IV center. Matter of fact, they were in town before we were. Well, the IV place went out of business, and he considered absorbing it.

He's a great marketer, he's a smart guy, and he works his butt off. So, he thought about it and realized "this isn't really my thing". Smart. We've had the chance to do cryo in our place, but we don't know anything about it. We could make money doing it, but we might eventually turn someone into a popsicle.

You might be fine getting an IV from the "we'll do anything we can make money on" place, but in our opinion you're always better sticking with an organization that specializes in one thing, and concentrates on doing it better than everyone else.

If they've got massage, cryotherapy, IVs, Botox, laser-derm abrasion, infrared something or other, Plasma Rich Platelet therapy and hormone replacement, are they really the best IV people in town?

8)   Budget environment

Straight honesty: when we started off we weren't in the nicest place. Matter of fact, it was just plain awful. The office itself was fine because we remodeled it by hand. We painted the walls ourselves, changed out all the light switches and electric outlet covers, and on and on and on. One thing we didn't skimp on was the medical end of things.

If an IV center is in a budget building, with budget furniture, doesn't have their own logo shirts/scrubs and such as that, what else are the choosing to go budget with? You don't want one that was so strapped financially they might decide to use an IV they mixed this morning that the patient decided not to get. You don't want one that opened a package of tubing, didn't use it, set it on a counter, and decided to use it on you because they couldn't afford to throw away 5 bucks worth of supplies.

All startups that are on a budget aren't cutting corners, but all other things being equal, why risk it?

9)   "Anything Goes" IV center

If you look at the "menu" for an IV center, and you see a bunch of things you don't recognize or understand, that might be a problem. ***Even if they're only doing IV therapy***, if they're doing every kind of questionable IV under the sun, whether it has been proven effective or not, be cautious.

In general, aside from the fact that as previously discussed it's hard to be great at a whole lot of different things, it indicates they're doing anything they think they can make money doing, whether it's a good idea or not.

The one we really see way more than we should (since we don't think we should see it in this setting at all), is ketamine. Why? Well, several reasons, but first and foremost is that the medical community just don't know enough about it.

Ketamine isn't Advil, or vitamins, or even Prozac, it's a serious anesthetic. SERIOUS. Though there's plenty of reading about it available online, about all you need to know is the first sentence from Wikipedia:

"Ketamine is a medication mainly used for starting and maintaining anesthesia. It induces a trance-like state while providing pain relief, sedation, and **memory loss**."

It's anesthesia. That induces memory loss. A lot of people nationwide are using it for depression or pain-relief, or any number of other things, but there's a reason they have to have crash carts sitting around when you get it.

IV Ketamine clinics are popping up all over the country and they're highly profitable, but you know what we like more than vacation homes and boats? Our patients. We're sure there are people doing these infusions safely, but there's just too much risk, from cardiac distress to pulmonary insufficiency to potential addiction and more, and not enough good science about why it should be used and how it can be used safely, in it for our taste.

You can't do it without a Nurse Anesthetist or Anesthesiologist present in the room when it's given, and they have to have a defibrillator (that gadget that restarts your heart) and crash cart handy. The simple fact that the FDA realizes there's a good enough chance you're going to crash that they require a crash cart is enough to scare us away.

If you want to read more, from the real experts, check out a publication from the American Psychiatric Association at https://psychnews.psychiatryonline.org/doi/full/10.1176/appi.pn.2018.pp1b1

I guess if you can't remember why you were depressed, that's something, but are you willing to be anesthetized next to a crash cart because you're a little down? Think three times about this one.

Honestly, I'm pretty damned near certain that the FDA is going to shut this down (outside of a hospital environment) sooner rather than later.

9) "That" doctor

I'm going to get roasted for this, but not by you, and you're why I wrote this book.

I've grown up with and around doctors (Dad, two uncles, Grandpa), work for and with doctors (still to this day), and have the utmost respect for the profession. That said, there are some physicians who want to do anything their license will allow them to do, other than be a "physician".

In more than one city where we have locations there are real-live medical doctors who run half-cocked alternative practices that do every last thing they can make a dollar on that doesn't include a legit annual wellness exam, a prostate exam, an

EKG, a complete blood count, or any of the real reasons you go see a "doc"-"tor".

Here's a list for you from one of these "Alt-Health-O-Rama Doc" places, which actually lists ALL of these things as "specialties". Keep in mind, if you've got more than a few "specialties", NONE of them are "specialties":

Sexual Health
Women's Health
Pain Management
Mental Health
Longevity and Regenerative Medicine
IV Therapy – NEW! (ding, ding, ding)
Immune Health
Men's Health
Beauty and Aesthetics
Weight Loss and Detox
Chronic Conditions
Hormone Health

So there you have it. Every last thing that a medical license will allow you to do that isn't really being a doctor. They've got more weird laser, heat wrap, electro-stimulus, and ultrasound machines than a research and development center.

When you walk into this person's office you can rest assured that someone really is an expert... at finding ways to make a buck. Unless you're Houston Methodist and have 100 employees at a location, each of whom ONLY does one thing, there's just no damned way these people know what they're doing. They don't even know why you're there when you walk in. Looking for hormones, lip injections, anti-aging voodoo medicines, weight loss laser-wrappers, or maybe an IV...

You've found a doctor who wants to sit in an office while a bunch of nurses, aestheticians, and mid-levels administer anything they think is profitable. I once knew a doctor, a really good one actually until he reached the end of his career and didn't want to "work" anymore, who bought two expensive "lose weight with this electronic treatment" machines. I can't say the name or I'll get sued. Anyway, I asked him if it really worked, because honestly, I could shed a few myself. He said "hell no, but people want it and think it does, and they advertise the hell out of it, so I might as well make money on it."

It may be that a doctor is very "new age" and tries all sorts of "off the beaten path" remedies, but the odds are that you're dealing with someone who couldn't make it in a regular office medical practice because the patients simply didn't knock down the doors, is tired of doctoring, or just isn't that great at being a doctor. Not your best bet.

CHAPTER 8:

Why Won't Insurance Pay For an IV in This Setting?

There's a bit of a misconception around this topic. Most people think that because you can't use your Blue Cross card at the IV center down on the corner there's something "sketchy" about the whole process.

You'll probably be surprised to hear it, but the vast majority of the time the fact that you can't use your insurance at an IV center isn't a decision made by Blue Cross (or United, or Cigna, Humana, et al), it's a decision made by the IV center.

Now you might be wondering why the hell any medical facility would decline to accept insurance.

Have you ever had a sleep study, an MRI, a CPAP, or been referred to a specialist by your primary care doctor? If you have, you know you didn't walk in the same day… or the next day… or the day after.

Any time you are referred for a service, the insurance company requires what's called a "prior authorization". Those can take days. When you need an IV, whether it's for a migraine, a hangover, dehydration, or food poisoning, you don't have two days to wait. After you've suffered for two days, it's over. You missed a party, your kid's game, and felt like hell for 48 hours, but it's over. No point in getting an IV Tuesday for food poisoning Sunday morning.

If you don't have authorization, the insurance company just slaps you with the entire bill. That's where it gets really tricky. The "allowed charge" that most insurance companies attach to a typical IV center treatment is MUCH higher than what you'd be charged at the facility if you paid cash.

Even IF you got an immediate authorization, or your insurance company didn't require one, it's likely that your deductible and/or co-pay would be more than the IV center would charge you cash.

You've probably seen crazy ER bills for IVs that run thousands and thousands of dollars. The last I saw was $3,600 for the same thing for which we (Rapid Recovery) charge $169.

Let's say you haven't met your deductible for the year, and your deductible is $2,500. Well, you're going to pay the first $2,500, and 80% of the remaining $1,100 ($220), for a whopping $2,720.

Even if you HAVE met your deductible you're going to pay 20% of the $3,600 charge, for a smooth $720.

How can that be? Well, ERs have to pay an orthopedic trauma surgeon to be on-call every night. They have to pay a cardiologist to be on-call. They generally have a pulmonologist/critical care doctor on call. They always have a whole staff of nurses. Those people don't come cheap.

Hospitals aren't gouging you. Their profit margin isn't great. If a hospital hits a 7% margin, it's knocking it out of the park. The problem is that they give a lot of care that isn't paid for (people coming into the ER and never paying, for example), and they have to have massive amounts of expensive staff to be able to cover all contingencies. That's why an Advil shows up on your bill at $58. You aren't paying $58 for the Advil, you're paying $58 for the lights to be on at the hospital when you show up with a heart attack.

An IV center doesn't have those issues. They pay a lease, they pay a small staff, they pay for snacks and drinks and medicine and supplies, but that's about it... so, they can charge you a hundred and fifty bucks and still earn a living.

A bit of good news is that because every IV is given (at least at reputable centers) only by prescription, you can generally pay for them with HSA and FSA cards. If your chosen center doesn't accept HAS or FSA cards, ask them if they are actually generating a prescription for your IV. If they don't have a script for every IV, you might not be at the right place.

CHAPTER 10:

How Often Can I Get an IV

Slow down cowpoke. The questions (in this order) should be "how often is it *safe* to get an IV" and "how often will I *need* an IV".

Remember, an IV in this setting should generally be an "oops" situation. "Ooops, stayed out in the sun too long." "Ooops, had a few too many." "Ooops, shouldn't have hugged little Billy when I knew he was sick."

Some people might need to regularly stop by an IV place. Runners who don't alter their schedule when the weather turns hot might be regulars. Business travelers who don't have the time to eat right might get a regular IV. Certainly, if you work outside in roofing, oil and gas, HVAC, or landscaping, you're going to be dehydrated more often than you aren't, and it's okay for you to swing by weekly. Some people with chronic illnesses have a reason to come fairly often.

If, however, you don't have a good reason to come weekly, don't. You'll simply pass the majority of what you're given (other than the fluids) in your urine.

So, back to that "how often is it safe to get an IV" question.

It depends entirely on what you're getting in those IVs. Actually, before I continue, let me say something about scheming the system. The good centers will have a limit on how often you can get certain IVs. DO NOT be the person who gets an IV at Place A, calls Place A in 3 days to ask for another and gets told "not for two more days", and then goes to Place B because they don't know you just went to Place A. There's a reason these places have rules and limitations. They're for your safety. No matter what you think you know, this is what these people do for a living and they know what's safe, and what isn't. Please don't be the person who tries to skirt around the rules. You could end up really getting hurt and risking someone's medical license.

Now, back to "what's in the IV", and how what's in them affects the safety of getting one.

If you're getting an IV with ketorolac (or basically any pain reliever) in it, you need to remember that stuff processes through your liver. Even though you're getting a liter of fluids to help keep it from damaging you, you can't keep getting NSAIDs via IV unless you eventually want to turn your liver into oatmeal.

Let's say you're getting Vitamin C via IV, and you are going to a place that's more concerned with making money than doing the right thing for its patients, or you're going from one to another to cheat the limits. Did you know that routinely getting more than 2 grams of Vitamin C can absolutely wreck your digestive system? You can quickly end up with diarrhea, acid reflux, and wicked nausea. Some people have been diagnosed with GI bleeds after continuous over-use of Vitamin C.

Vitamin D over and over and over again can be just as bad or worse. Not only do you get the nausea, vomiting, and diarrhea, you can end up with hypercalcemia (remember, D aids in the absorption of calcium), and that can lead to serious cardiac issues. If you're lucky you'll just get kidney stones from the hypercalcemia. If you aren't lucky, you get heart problems.

So, don't ask "how often **CAN** I get an IV", ask "how often **SHOULD** I get an IV". Just as importantly, ask someone who cares more about you as a person than they do about your credit card.

An honest IV center will tell you something like "that's great Jane, and we love having you here, but you should wait til next week for another one of those IVs."

It's really hard to do that as an IV center, because the people who want to come all the time are the people who keep the lights on, but the right thing to do is tell the truth and put the electric bill on a credit card, because eventually doing the right thing for the patient pays off in the long run. Find that place, and you've got a winner.

CHAPTER 11:

Where Do I Get an IV?

Well, we've discussed this in general terms, and we'll go over it here again briefly, and then we'll get specific.

First: Look for a place that is specific to IVs. With few exceptions, the places that specialize in something are better at it. An Audi-specific mechanic probably knows Audis better than the guy at a place called "We Fix All Cars".

Second: Pick a place that mixes its own IVs. If you don't, you'll either get something you don't need, don't want, or shouldn't have. Custom is always better.

Third: Make sure it's clean and tidy.

Fourth: Make sure they have all the proper certifications and licenses.

Five: Check the reviews.

So, now that you know these things, where specifically would I send you? Well, by city, here's where I'm comfortable sending you:

Allen, Texas - InfusaLounge

There is no harder worker in the IV industry, not even us, than Melissa Chester. If it's good she wants it better, if it's great she wants it the best. Just knowing how hard she works at InfusaLounge is tiring.

Charlotte, North Carolina - Hydrate Medical

Run by one of the most well respected ER docs I know. Doesn't let anything slip through the cracks, and is happy to share his knowledge. Policies are exemplary. Hydrate is now opening their SIXTH location. They've exploded, and rapidly, because Dr. Jonathan Leake is a relentlessly driven professional who created a system that's known for quality.

Chicago, Illinois - IVme

One of the originals, and still one of the best. I believe IVme was the third IV center in the country, and they have taken to their role of being "leaders" in the industry. They have a stellar clinical staff. Dr. Jack Dybis is interviewed in every publication in the country because he's known as "the hydration guru". His partner Scott Yilk is a super human being and is incredibly hands-on. Ask for Gina by the way. So good. So cool. One of the best nurses you'll ever meet.

I'll let you in on a secret. One of our nurses was running the Chicago Marathon, and do you know what we did? We paid for her to go to IVme. That's how much we trust what they do.

Colorado Springs, Colorado - Elevation Hydration

The single best IV starter I've ever seen or heard about. If I found myself in the back of an ambulance and only had one shot at someone hitting my vein, there's zero question in my mind that Corey Garrett Brown is the person I'd pick. You generally can't tell who is the "best ___ in the country", whether it's a baseball player or a restaurant, or whatever, because there are so many people who are great at what they do, but I'm pretty confident that Corey is actually the BEST IV starter in the country. I don't know any in other countries so I'll just stop at the borders.

If you go to Elevation Hydration and they don't do a great job, I'll give you back the money you spent on this book. If all IV centers were as good at starting IVs as Elevation Hydration, nobody would be afraid to get an IV. We actually took a trip to learn from them, and it has paid off handsomely.

Dallas, Texas - Vitalogy

There's a reason they already have four locations. Innovation. One step ahead at all times. The owner, Todd Wesson, consistently tracks down information and ideas to try to perfect his craft, and has partnered with pharmacies to provide very custom mixes.

Denver, Colorado - Hydrate IV Bar

Best reviews on the web. I was afraid of them initially (before I got to know their quality) because of the name, but they're very professional, and Katie, the owner, works her butt off to keep her patients happy. They've got three or more locations by now because people in the Mile High City absolutely trust her to always do the right thing.

El Paso, Texas - Drip Drive

Ashley Nahle is the most loved owner of any IV spa I know. Even other IV spa owners who compete with her love Ashley. Her employees love her. Her patients love her. She's just a genuinely caring human being who really simply wants everyone to feel better. You'll love her too.

Milwaukee, Wisconsin - Health Hydration Oasis

H_2O gets my vote for best medical director/owner, ANYWHERE. Dr. Alia Fox has H_2O so far above and beyond what's required, they don't even remember what the "required line" is. Regulations are what everyone else strives to meet. Dr. Fox would cringe if H_2O only met the regulations. Actually, if she wrote the IV spa regulations all the IV centers would be better.

When Dr. Fox isn't anesthetizing surgical patients in a local hospital, or sitting at a charity organization's board meeting, she's in one of her locations checking to make sure everything is going according to plan, and she might even start an IV or two.

Just as an aside, if Gloria Vanderbilt were still alive, even she would be impressed by the décor in H2O. Plus Dr. Fox is an awarded anesthesiologist, has a list of celebrity patients a mile long, and looks like a model. Don't you hate people like that? ;-)

New Orleans, Louisiana - Remedy Room

The Founder/Resident Physician (Mignonne Mary, M.D.) is not just an IV star, she's a wellness GURU. Actually, it's pretty widely thought that her father was the originator of IV therapy as we know it today.

Dr. Mary is as dedicated to your health as... well, she might be more dedicated to your health than you are. She and her staff don't just do IVs, they do videos to help you eat right, breathe right, exercise, fast when appropriate... it's endless. More importantly, it's not all about getting you to buy an injection or an IV from Remedy Room, she just genuinely wants you to be healthy.

Odessa, Texas - Enliven

Katrina Bustos is the owner, and she's simply relentless about learning, improving, and doing anything she can to be better. For the past several years we've consistently watched her spend hour after hour researching best practices, best medicines, best procedures, and trying to improve Enliven. It's very impressive.

We own **Rapid Recovery**, an IV center with locations in **Shreveport, Louisiana, Tyler, Texas, and Sunnyvale (Mesquite/East Dallas), Texas**, and we like to think we do a great job. Of course we would though, so check out our reviews, troll our website (https://www.RapidRecoveryRoom. com), ask to see our Policies and Procedures, and pick up the phone to talk to us. That's always good practice for any IV center you want to use.

There are probably dozens, if not hundreds, of others, but those are the ones with which I'm familiar and for which I'm comfortable vouching. When our patients or family are out of town, those are the places I send them, with full confidence.

CHAPTER 12:

Summing It All Up

IV therapy is a great addition to your healthcare regimen, and fantastic in a pinch. It's wonderful for dehydration, jet lag, recovering from illness, stopping a migraine or hangover in its tracks, feeling better after chemo, and dozens of other things.

It's not a miracle cure, and it isn't going to take years off your looks. It isn't going to cure cancer or keep you from getting (or looking) older.

Go to a reputable IV center that focuses on IVs and doesn't also offer every BS wellness treatment under the sun, follows solid policies and procedures, has an involved physician of an appropriate specialty, asks a lot of questions, qualifies you physically for the IV, and takes care of you after the IV is done.

Most importantly, ASK. If you're worried about something, ask. If you don't get the answer you want, or the person who answers doesn't appear confident or complete in their answer, walk out. Remember, this is about your health. There's no reason to get an IV unless you're comfortable.

An IV, of the right type, in the right place, at the right time, can really help you feel better faster. Do your homework, then relax and enjoy.

Thanks for reading. I hope something in here helped you. If you have any questions, you've got my email. If you don't have it, wheeler@rapidrecoveryroom.com will do.

WITH SPECIAL THANKS TO:

Rachel for believing it could happen and working for free,

Emma for driving all over Hell and half the ArkLaTex with us,

Mom and Dad for the usual "everything" thing,

Bert for giving me the time off to pursue a goal,

Evan Stanley with McKesson for going above and beyond to make sure we always have what we need, and being way more than a "vendor",

Dr. Shaik for being patient, concerned, enthusiastic, and involved,

Corey Garrett Brown for being an unrelenting source of ideas, inspiration, faith, and positivity, and a damned good friend,

Don Zimmerman for being the best radio guy I've ever known and doing everything he can to help us grow,

All of our Facebook family, email subscribers, blog readers, and followers,

Alia Fox, Gina Werner, Scott Yilk, Jonathan Leake, Melissa Chester, Katrina Bustos, Heather Kessler, and Ashley Nahle for all the advice, help, and encouragement,

Timbo Reid of the Small Business Big Marketing Show, for teaching us (among countless thousands of others) how to take our baby from a struggling little business to a thriving enterprise, motivating us to take action, and (quite confusingly) never asking a penny for the wisdom,

Our nurses, who really are the best in the business and make it easy to sleep at night,

and most of all, those folks who have come to see us for an IV or injection, counted on us to help them Feel Better Faster, and trusted us to take care of them over the last five years.